Mastering the DSM-5

Implementing New Measures and Assessments in Your Clinical Practice

By Mary L. Flett, Ph.D.

"This is the only work I've seen that addresses the complexity of Section Three in the DSM 5® with clarity, details and examples for its application. Dr. Flett has given us a valuable adjunct to the DSM® which will enhance diagnostics and clarify levels of distress and disability. This book should be considered a must in understanding the DSM 5®."

-Jack Klott, MSSA, LISW, CSW & national DSM-5® speaker & expert

Copyright © 2014 by Mary L. Flett, Ph.D.

Published by
PESI Publishing & Media
PESI, Inc
3839 White Ave
Eau Claire, WI 54703

Printed in the United States of America

ISBN: 978-1-937661-41-0

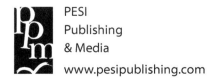

PESI
Publishing
& Media
www.pesipublishing.com

Dedication

To my husband, for seeing in me the things I could not see for myself; to my teachers, for helping me develop the skills and discipline to think and write; and to my clients, for being willing to open up and share.

Table of Contents

About the Author

Mary L. Flett, Ph.D., is a respected national speaker on the DSM-5 and how it is revolutionizing diagnosis and treatment. She is a licensed psychologist who focuses her practice on aging issues and behavioral rehabilitation, partnering with medical professionals, integrative medicine practitioners, and complimentary healing providers. Dr. Flett has worked in private practice, community-based agencies, and has provided services in both state and county government behavioral health systems. In addition to her clinical work across the developmental spectrum, Dr. Flett has conducted evaluation and outcomes analyses and quality improvement studies for county and state government. She has also taught at both the undergraduate and graduate levels.

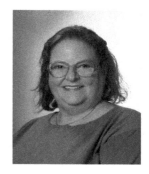

Preface

This book will give you step-by-step instructions on how you can integrate the measures and evaluation tools contained in the DSM-5® and use them to inform your work with your clients and with others who interact with your clients.

A word about terms in this book: As a psychologist, I frequently switch between calling the individuals I work with "clients", "consumers", or "patients". The change-up comes from having been in the field for over 20 years and also from the differences in nomenclature between professions.

I appreciate consistency as much as being politically correct. Use of language that is sensitive to the impact it has on those reading and listening and participating is something I have spent time considering in writing this book. I have intentionally chosen to use the word "client" throughout. It makes for consistent reading and understanding. I do not want you, the reader, to be distracted from what I am trying to say, nor do I want you thinking that I am adopting language reflective of pejorative applications of our work.

Introduction

WHY USE ASSESSMENT MEASURES IN MENTAL HEALTH?

Although this seems an obvious question with an obvious answer, it is useful to clarify at the start what benefits there are to using assessment measures that have met standards of evidence-based practice. Just as you would not use a ruler to determine how much a person weighs, the use of the appropriate and accurate measurement makes a difference both in how information is gathered and the meaning that can be made of the results for individuals with mental disorders.

I believe it is useful to use assessment measures to see if what I am doing is making a difference in my client's life. I also believe that it is useful to my client to see that I am monitoring our work and that progress is being made. Finally, I believe it is useful to share results with my clients so that they see how our working together is making a difference in their lives.

Assessments are frequently used to gather information for other purposes such as program evaluation and/or justifying or confirming benefit for grants. It is important in situations like this that the findings be made useful to all stakeholders—staff, consumers, students, grant funders, etc. Without useful information, the administration of the measures can frequently be seen as a barrier or worse, a form of punishment that gets in the way of the therapeutic connection needed to create opportunities for change.

Having a positive, open attitude toward implementation of these measures is key in assuring that the benefits and value of the effort needed are sustained. Development of this attitude comes from exposure to the measures themselves, allowing for adequate training and understanding of how the measures can be used, and a thorough immersion in the scoring and interpretation of the results. Only at that point can the clinician begin to make meaning of the results in collaboration with the client.

Too often there is a gap between the need for data and how it is gathered. What seems to be missing is letting all the participants in on the "Why?" I have worked in a variety of settings where these aspirational values have not been achieved, resulting in resentment by clinicians, frustration by clients, and a waste of valuable time on the part of administrators and supervisors across specialties.

My experience has opened my eyes to the necessity of finding ways for clinicians to apply the information gathered using these measures both to impact the work with clients, and to shift the focus from "getting the information" to "using the results". Depending on your setting (private practice, clinic, government, military), how you incorporate these tools will provide you with opportunities to learn more about how you practice, how your clients/respond to your approach, and how the systems you interact with can be improved. And this does not need to be burdensome, onerous, or a barrier to your doing your work the way you do it.

The fact that you are picking up this book suggests that you already have some ideas about the use of behavioral measurements. My goal in the remainder of this book is to share some of my ideas, having worked with and struggled to find practical uses for measures such as these, and to show you ways to integrate these tools into your practice. Whether you are an experienced clinician, researcher, program evaluator, or a graduate student, this book will clearly explain the measures, provide examples of how they can be used in a variety of practice settings, and inspire you to use them in improving your work.

HOW TO USE THIS BOOK

This book is designed so that you can go to a specific chapter discussing one measure, get an overview of its development and how it can be used, and how to score, interpret, and apply that information to your practice. You can also start at the beginning and just move through each chapter.

You can use this book as a resource for forms and interpretive guidelines when administering the measures. Each chapter includes information on how to explore the results and make meaning with your clients and with other treatment professionals.

Finally, you can use this book as an adjunct to the DSM-5.

PLANNING FOR CHANGE

How do you get started? This takes a bit of planning and thought, but it follows a well-established format. This is known as continuous quality improvement and has four basic phases: plan, do, study, act. The steps are identified below. Resources for implementing change in various settings are discussed in the following chapters.

The first phase is usually the most time-consuming, and possibly frustrating, because we are more inclined to want to "do" than to "plan". Once a plan is in place, however, the "doing" follows naturally. But if the process stops there, it will most likely result in little or no gain because there has been no opportunity to do the metacognition necessary to evaluate what the "doing" has accomplished. The third phase, "study", oftentimes is simultaneous with the doing. The final phase, "act" implies that changes and/or modifications are made and implemented. Just how long this process takes is entirely dependent upon who is "on-board" and how specific you are in your goals. Vague goals typically result in vague outcomes.

You may find that some of the measures and assessments are more useful or more applicable to your practice than others. This is not an 'all-or-nothing' proposition. Each of the measures is in the public domain. There are other, similar instruments available for purchase from psychological assessment companies that you can use if you have been trained and meet the qualifications for administration, scoring and interpretation. These assessments and measures differ across license, scope of practice, and state and federal regulations. Taking some time to look at the instruments provided in the DSM-5 and on the DSM-5 website, understanding how they were developed, and who their intended audience is, will help you to select those that meet your needs, and the needs of your clients.

Scoring and interpretation of the results is not self-evident. While administration is fairly straightforward, the scoring of some of the instruments is complex and needs some set-up. Additionally, the interpretation of the results also needs time and attention so that you can understand and effectively share the implications of the results with your clients.

None of these measures is designed to diagnose in and of itself; rather each is designed to elicit information that will inform you so that you can arrive at a diagnosis using all your skills, experience, and training. Measurement is an art as well as a science. It requires attention to detail and solid clinical judgment. Your ability to infer and interpret results will improve with each administration.

CHAPTER 1

Implementing Change

With the publication of the DSM-5, for the first time practitioners are provided with tools specifically developed for use with the manual. While there is no requirement that these tools be used, a clear signal is being sent that measuring change is going to be part of how practitioners are expected to practice. Depending on your level of training, you may have had extensive exposure to the use of assessments and measures in determining diagnosis and informing treatment plans. Or, perhaps you only had a class or two and have never considered using measures such as the WHODAS 2.0 or the Level-1 Cross-Cutting Symptom Measures as part of your intake, evaluation, and treatment plan.

If you fit into the latter category, it is important that you familiarize yourself with the challenges of implementing these tools in your practice, whether it be as a solo practitioner, someone who works in an agency or group, or who works with several different systems. It is also important that you understand the limitations of these tools, as well as their applications.

The DSM-5 does not provide training or support in using these tools. That is the focus of this book.

Getting Started

How do you get started incorporating assessment measures into your practice? As noted above, this takes a bit of planning and thought, but follows the well-established format of continuous quality improvement: plan, do, study, act.

Phase I: Planning for Change

Planning will address several different areas depending on how you practice. If you are a sole practitioner, it may include determining which of the measures fits your practice profile. For example, you may wish to use the WHODAS 2.0

and the Level 1 Cross-Cutting Symptoms for all your clients, or maybe just some. You will also need to decide when you want to begin using these measures. Will you begin using them only for new clients or will you ask current clients to complete the measures? How will you share the results? How will you track when you re-administer the measures? An implementation checklist for private practice is provided in Appendix B.

If you are working in an agency or a group, you will need to get buy-in from your colleagues. Additionally, you (or someone) will need to review policies and procedures related to gathering information. This can be time-consuming, but it will pay off in the end. Having alignment between policy and practice is essential to insuring the success of implementing change. The balance of the planning stage mirrors that found for private practitioners. You will need to add in training on the instruments, and determine who will do the scoring and interpretation.

System Flow of Information

Since there are more individuals who will be involved in "touching" the information, you will need to identify how this information flows through the system. For example, while the clinician may administer the measure, there may be another individual who bills for the time, another individual who collects the data, another individual who scores and produces the results, and several other individuals who review the chart. Systematically identifying everyone who "touches" the data and determining their responsibility for managing that information is necessary in insuring there are no data drops or gaps in the system.

Many people are now using computerized systems to gather information. You may need additional code written for incorporating forms into electronic health records (EHR) and uploading results. Policies need to be reviewed to insure that they are consistent with the administration needs for these measures, specifically regarding qualifications of who can and cannot administer, score, and interpret the results.

Training

Training of staff on how to administer, score, and interpret the results will need to be done. Planning for this would include all current staff as appropriate, and any new staff who come on board after this process is implemented. Handbooks and/or guidelines will need to be written, if that is usual for the agency or practice. It is always prudent to have written policies and handbooks to document the purpose and use of this information whether you are a sole practitioner or working in an agency or group.

Costs

While the measures are free, there are a number of costs associated with implementing them. As noted above, computer code may need to be written, staff will need to be trained, and training materials created and provided. Costs for reproducing the materials (unless downloaded each time from APA) are also a consideration. Budgeting for these and other ancillary costs should be part of the planning process.

Who Should Be Involved in Planning?

Depending on the configuration of your agency or group, key individuals who should be involved include clinicians, finance staff, computer programmers, quality improvement staff, supervisors, training staff, coders/billers, chartroom personnel, and stakeholders. More information on this can be found in Chapter 7.

Time Frame

Planning when to implement the change is important. You will need to take into consideration new clients, and former clients who may come back. You will need to think about 'grandfathering' in current clients. Setting a "date certain" is a useful strategy. That way, everyone will know when the process is going to start and how to address current, new, and former clients. In my own practice, I put a note in each chart when I began using the measures. This went into every chart, even the ones where I did not actually provide a measure. That way, when I open the chart up, I know where I stand. This is a more challenging aspect of implementation when working in an agency or group.

PHASE 2: "DO"

This is actually more like a shake-down cruise than an actual implementation. In implementing this in my private practice, I made several false starts before I found a way to incorporate these measures that was consistent with the way I practice and met the needs of my clients. Expecting there to be glitches and problems is actually the most realistic way to approach this phase.

In an agency or group setting, you would most likely want to do at least one pilot before actually implementing the process full-on. The pilot would probably consist of your most enthusiastic users and one or two folks who are not supporters. That way you can get a feel for what may actually occur. Having buy-in here is crucial.

Give the pilot a reasonable amount of time and a reasonable number of clients so that the information you gather is representative of what may actually happen. Use this information to make adaptations to the process. You may need to do several pilots in order to maximize your data gathering and save money on full implementation. The advice here is: "Be Patient". It will save you money and good will in the long run.

PHASE 3: STUDY

The third phase, "study", oftentimes is simultaneous with "doing." In my own practice, I noticed that there were several parts of the process that needed adjustment. I only learned this after actually administering these measures to several different clients over the period of several months. My first discovery was that I couldn't just give the measures to the client and expect them to read through the questions and bring it back to me. I had to explain what the measures were for and what information I hoped to get from them. Then I had to think about how I would share the results. I tried several different ways until I determined that I would create charts that descriptively explained the results. This is what I finally settled on and am now using regularly. I have provided Excel spreadsheets with scoring and interpretive guidelines for the WHODAS and the Level-1 Cross-Cutting Symptoms in the Forms section.

Because this was being done simultaneously with my other clients, I needed to go back to the first set of folks I had used the measures with and ask them to respond again. This resulted in some new information, as well as confirming that the process I finally arrived at was going to be the one I would use.

The study phase in an agency or group should be a collaborative experience. All participants (including stakeholders) should be able to share their experiences and insights and then contribute to streamlining the process so that it actually accomplishes what it sets out to do: provide the clinician and client with useful information for treatment planning and interventions. It may be obvious, but it is worth stating; if only one individual (or a small group) interprets the results and then hands down a protocol, the buy-in from the rest of the group is likely to be small, and the effort will result in poor implementation or worse.

Getting Buy-In Using QFocus

A wonderful process to use in this stage is something called the "QFocus Technique" (Rothstein & Santana, 2012). I encourage you to visit the Right

Question website (http://rightquestion.org/make-just-one-change) to become more familiar with this process. I present it below in brief, modified for use in an agency or group practice. The process can take as little as 30 minutes if the group is cohesive and the facilitator has thought through what the QFocus question is. This is true even in a large group. I have used this process in a number of different settings and generally find that the median time for the process is closer to 45 minutes.

The process is designed to access and integrate divergent thinking, convergent thinking and metacognitive thinking skills. It is done in a group setting with a facilitator and small groups. The facilitator provides encouragement and guidance, but does not direct or interpret. The small groups increase the intensity of the thinking and the larger group incorporates the metacognition and conclusions reached. The process is found in Appendix A.

PHASE 4: ACT

The final phase, "act" implies that changes and/or modifications are made and implemented. Just how long this process takes is entirely dependent on who is on-board and how specific you are in your goals. Vague goals typically result in vague outcomes. If you use the QFocus process described in Appendix A, you may find that the last step actually creates the blueprint for implementation. If you use another process, you would want to come up with both "next steps" and assignment of responsibilities for accomplishing the implementation.

To achieve a positive result, you might want to follow this slightly modified CQI plan. 1) take the time to get the buy-in from all stakeholders and participants; 2) try a pilot first to see where unexpected problems lie; 3) collaborate on fixes and approaches; 4) take what you've learned and set a target implementation date; 5) Monitor to see how things are going; 6) share results and make necessary changes.

SHARING THE INFORMATION WITH YOUR CLIENTS

To make this information gathering process complete, it is important we share the information with our clients. But what does that mean? Do we just give them back their measures? Well, you could, but I want to suggest that you make the sharing of information a part of the CQI process, as part of the 'study' phase. This is where the meaning of the results emerges. The measure itself, unlike the Oracle at Delphi, does not tell "truth" – it merely reflects back, in an organized way, what the individual who completed it said on a particular day at a particular time in their lives. This is an important point to contemplate.

Depending on when you take a look at it, things may have changed dramatically or hardly changed at all. These are entrées into your client's world. Use them as passports to gain access, then explore how your clients function and think.

This process fits in nicely with the case conceptualization portion of your diagnosis and treatment planning. Based on what is uncovered, and the meaning your client ascribes to this, you can then go about tailoring your treatment plan to address the issues, while measuring the change.

Measurement of change typically consists of re-administering the instrument at several different points. Each of the instruments in the DSM-5 has good test-retest reliability, which means you can administer them again and again and the responses will provide useful information. *When* you decide to administer the instruments depends on several factors including how frequently you see the client, what levels of variability in change are expected, and your client's capacity to complete the instruments. It is a good idea to establish a baseline measurement, which is typically done at intake or shortly thereafter. You can then decide if you want to monitor based on symptom change or at regular intervals. Finally, completing a discharge evaluation, if possible, is also useful.

AM I GETTING BETTER?

One of the unstated effects of using measures is that both the client and the clinician may assume that these are measures of *improvement*. That is not the case. These are indicators of change. This may seem a fine point, but it is an important one to grasp. Change can be interpreted in many ways. If you have a fever and your temperature is going down, that is an indicator that your body is returning to normal. If you are underweight and you eat more calories and you step on the scale and the numbers go up, that is an indicator that you are putting on weight.

Indicators of Change

In the realm of DSM-5 measures, indicators include levels of distress (none to severe), numbers of symptoms (the more symptoms, the more likely impairment exists), domains of impairment (cognition, communication, self-care, participation in society), and experiences of culture. These do not lend themselves to quantitative measurement, thus they should not be considered measures of "progress" or "getting better", but indicators of where to begin and directionality (moving toward or away from). To assess that, these indicators are given numeric equivalents that can be used to detect change.

For example, the Likert scale used in the Level 1 Cross-Cutting Symptom Measure consists of "None", "Slight", "Mild", "Moderate", and "Severe". The numeric equivalents are 0, 1, 2, 3, and 4. Baseline measures of the symptoms consist of identifying the highest domain score as well as the total number of domains that have scores above 1. Directionality is determined by comparing the baseline scores within domains, and the total number of domains with scores above 1 with subsequent administrations. If the following administrations show a reduction in either number of domains impacted and/or lowering of the scores, then the indication is that the client's experience of distress is diminishing.

If the scores are not going down, or the total number of clusters impacted remains high, you can explore several different hypotheses. Perhaps there are situational variables (poverty, stress, environmental catastrophe) that can't be addressed through therapy alone, or perhaps there are contributing issues that haven't been identified, or perhaps the intervention and/or treatment is ineffective. When the variables are identified, you can then use the measures to see if the adjustments you have made are effective.

CONCLUSION

Making the decision to incorporate these new tools into your practice is just the start. How you decide to do this will take some advance planning, whether you are in private practice or in an agency or group setting. If you take the time to do this intentionally, I believe you will find the benefits are useful and practical. Making measurement a regular part of your practice will impact your clients in many positive ways. It will give them a voice in their process, it will give you insight into their experience, and it will provide you both with opportunities to reflect on what has been accomplished, where adjustments need to be made, and indicators for how those adjustments are working.

Be patient with the process.

CHAPTER 2

What in the World Is the WHODAS?

WORLD HEALTH ORGANIZATION DISABILITY ASSESSMENT SCHEDULE 2.0

In the DSM-III and IV, clinicians were asked to evaluate a client's functioning using the Global Assessment of Functioning (GAF). This is a 100-point scale that requires the clinician to provide a numeric point to describe the client's functioning. This was reported on Axis V, and completed the overall evaluation of the client.

While the concept of pinpointing functioning is useful, the GAF was inconsistently applied and often was incorporated as a summary of functioning rather than an evaluation of functioning. The WHODAS is a much richer, client-centered measure which has greater validity and reliability than the GAF. Using the WHODAS 2.0 retains the spirit of including functioning as a measure, and achieves an even higher standard of clinical utility.

INTRODUCTION

The WHODAS is a well-researched, well-tested instrument promulgated by the World Health Organization. Their website (http://www.who.int/en) is filled with interesting information about all types of issues, disability being only one amongst many. You can download the WHODAS training manual in pdf format from this website for more in-depth information on the development and application of this screen. I have summarized selected sections from the training manual below to give you a foundation from which to use this screening tool. With that said, I encourage the reader to obtain the training manual (especially since there is no charge!) and read through Chapter 7 which details how to administer and score the results. For those readers who may be working in a training setting with interns, there is a wonderful self-test in Chapter 10 on understanding the concepts fundamental to understanding the use and interpretation of the WHODAS 2.0.

9

The WHODAS 2.0 is a measure of general health that can be used for multiple purposes in different settings. This gives practitioners a great deal of flexibility in deciding with whom and how to use this information. There are three versions of the instrument, each discussed in more detail below. Each of these versions identifies issues within six domains of functioning, although each is done in a slightly different format.

Using the full version (36-items) of the assessment will provide clinicians with more specific information than the 12-item version. It may be useful to use the longer version, particularly if you are wanting to track changes over time. If you are more concerned with obtaining a general impression of how many areas of functioning are problematic, the more simple summary score will give you that information.

Self-Administered Version

A paper-and-pencil version containing 36 questions can be handed to clients and filled out by them. According to the training manual, "All questions share similar stems, and the same timeframe and response scale. This gives the instrument a user-friendly, uncluttered and to-the-point style." (Üstün, Kostanjsek, Chatterji, and Rehm, 2010, p. 37). This will most likely be the easiest and most common form for usage in most practice settings. The form is two pages long and can be downloaded from the WHODAS site in pdf format. There are no copyright restrictions.

Interview Format

Clinicians may choose to interview a client using the 12+24 question format, either due to limitations in the client (e.g., physical, situational, or educational deficits) or options available in the setting (e.g., phone interview or interview conducted by someone other than the clinician such as an intake coordinator). This format allows for a tiered evaluation whereby the initial questions asked can screen for levels of disability. Where none is reported, the interview is concluded, but, if the respondent reports levels of mild, moderate or severe, a second tier of questions is asked to further identify the issues.

Typical demographic and background data are gathered first, followed by a script that explains concepts such as "health condition", "difficulty with an activity", and degrees of impairment. Core questions are asked first to establish where and if there is functional disability at all. If there is none, the interview is concluded. If the client endorses any of the core questions with a degree of impairment greater than 'none', then an additional set of questions is asked. The final pass includes follow-up that is domain specific, again, based on the response of the client.

Proxy

The third approach is to use a proxy. This is useful where the client is unable or unwilling to share this information and/or where there may be discrepancies in statements between the client and other informants. It is also useful in gathering information from others such as caregivers, providers, or other observers. The proxy assessment is the same as the 12-question self-assessment except that it identifies the proxy as being husband or wife, parent, son or daughter, brother or sister, other relative, friend, professional caregiver, or other. It also includes a three-question screen for how many days the disability interfered with the individual's functioning.

You can give this to as many proxies as you feel would be useful. This can be invaluable information, particularly where there is a desire to include others in the care of the clients.

DEVELOPMENT OF THE **WHODAS**

If you have ever attempted to design a questionnaire, you will appreciate the challenges involved in developing one that reliably captures the information you want. The WHODAS was not developed for a single culture, it was developed to be used around the world, thus requiring even more rigorous and creative ways to accomplish this. According to the developers, methods used WHODAS included:

- a collaborative international approach, with the aim of developing a single generic instrument for assessing health status and disability in different settings;
- a unique set of cross-cultural applicability study protocols to ensure that WHODAS 2.0 would have a high degree of functional and metric equivalence across different cultures and settings; and
- a connection with the revision of the International Classification of Functioning (ICF), to allow the new instrument to be directly linked to the ICF (see http://www.who.int/classifications/icf/whodasii/en/index1.html).

Clinicians can rest assured that this instrument has undergone rigorous psychometric testing as well as being culturally sensitive. An added benefit is that culturally and linguistically appropriate translations of the instrument are available.

Clinicians can access translations on the WHODAS website for the following languages: Albanian, Arabic, Bengali, Chinese (Mandarin), Croatian, Czech, Danish, Dutch, English, Finnish, French, German, Greek, Hindi, Italian, Japanese, Kannada, Korean, Norwegian, Portuguese, Romanian, Russian, Serbian, Slovenian, Spanish, Sinhala, Swedish, Tamil, Thai, Turkish and Yoruba.

DESCRIPTION OF THE DOMAINS

The WHODAS 2.0 looks at functioning across six specific domains: cognition, mobility, self-care, getting along, life activities (household and work) and participation in society. Functioning is not assumed to be static, rather it is expected to change, and therefore it can be measured. The WHODAS will not tell you "why" someone is having problems functioning, but it will tell you which areas, if any, pose problems for the client.

The following description of each of the domains is intended to provide readers with a brief overview. Those who wish to explore the psychometric properties of the question sets within each domain should refer to the WHODAS training manual (Üstün, et al., 2010, pp. 48-50).

Cognition comprises questions about communication and thinking activities. Specific areas assessed include concentrating, remembering, problem solving, learning and communicating.

Mobility questions explore the client's ability to stand, move around inside the home, get out of the home and walk a long distance. The latter uses the term "kilometer", since the rest of the world uses the metric system.

Self-care looks at the client's ability to manage bathing, dressing, eating, and staying alone.

These first three areas are typically considered by most clinicians in evaluating how well a client functions. The addition of three other domains makes the WHODAS especially useful in assessing individuals with behavioral health issues (Üstün, et al., 2010, pp. 51-53).

Getting along assesses the client's ability to relate to other people, and explores difficulties that might be encountered with this due to a health condition. This may include intimates (e.g. spouse or partner, family members or close friends), or strangers.

Life activities includes activities that people do on most days such as household tasks, and attendance at work and school. The questions explore the client's difficulty in engaging in these activities on a day-to-day basis. Definitions for what each of these activities include are provided on a flashcard.

Participation asks clients to consider how other people and the world around them make it difficult for them to take part in society. The focus of these questions is on how the environment (external factors) as opposed to their own difficulties (internal factors) impacts their ability to function. This domain also includes questions about the impact of their health condition. "Here, they are reporting not on their activity limitations but rather on the restrictions they experience from people, laws and other features of the world in which they find themselves." (Üstün, Chatterji, Kostanjsek, & Rehm (2010), p. 61).

Information gathered from the WHODAS can be beneficial for beginning many conversations about the individual's world and how they manage their challenges. It is also useful in terms of monitoring change.

APPLICATIONS

One of the challenges of assessing functioning is finding a time period that is not too long and not too short. If it is too long, the variability can be lost. If it is too short, the variability may be missed all together. The WHODAS looks at functioning retrospectively over a period of 30 days. It asks clients to think about their functioning in terms of the degree of difficulty experienced ("none", "mild", "moderate", "severe", and "extreme or cannot do"). The term "functioning" refers to the problems encountered by the client because of their health condition, which includes physical, emotional, and substance use. These frames of reference are then weighed by asking the clients to average good and bad days.

The terms are very specifically defined. For example, "having difficulty" means requiring increased effort, experiencing discomfort or pain, involving slowness, and/or changes in the way the person does the activity. "Health conditions" includes things like diseases, illnesses or other health problems, injuries, mental or emotional problems, problems with alcohol, and problems with drugs. "Usual way of doing activity" includes adaptive devices and assistance. These examples are shared with the client to help them understand what is being assessed. The manual provides examples to illustrate these.

The focus of the WHODAS is on the amount of difficulty encountered in activities that the client actually does, as opposed to those s/he would like to or can do, but doesn't actually do. For example, if your client drives everywhere, s/he might answer the question about walking a mile as "N/A". But if your client has a broken leg, the same question would be answered "Extreme or cannot do". Or, a client who lives with family members might answer the question about ability to be alone for several days as "Cannot do" because s/he believes it would be difficult, whereas the appropriate answer would be "Not Applicable" because they weren't actually ever alone during the last 30 days.

Using the Information with Clients

The WHODAS is a self-report measure. This means the information should not be considered "accurate" or "right or wrong", rather it should be thought of qualitatively. In other words, use this assessment to obtain "feeling-based" responses, not "thinking-based". Responses given by the clients will reflect their perception of why they are being asked to complete this, as well as the administrator's bias for or against the instrument. Acknowledging this is particularly important if you are using the WHODAS in an institutional setting. If this is "just another thing to do" then the likelihood of obtaining useful responses may decrease. If staff and clients understand that this is a sincere attempt to gather information that will make a difference in the client's life, then the responses will reflect that sincerity.

Scoring the WHODAS

There are two ways to score the WHODAS. The first is to simply add all the answers together to obtain a total score. The higher the score, the greater the disability interferes with optimal functioning. It is likely that this method would be used in most clinical settings, as it is quick and easy. This will provide clinicians and clients with easily understood information that can be compared over time. It should not, however, be used to compare different populations.

A more elegant scoring of the WHODAS involves using item-response theory (IRT). The psychometric properties of the WHODAS are quite robust when it comes to internal consistency. Agencies may choose to use IRT to compare populations or as performance improvement indicators. Because IRT allows for more fine-grained analysis, the actual scoring is more complex. The generosity and spirit of true research is evident in that the editors of the WHODAS manual provide SPSS language for scoring each of the domains (Üstün, et al., 2010). For readers interested in using this level of analysis, you need only download the SPSS syntax at the WHO website.

WHAT DO THE SCORES MEAN?

It is important to remember that the WHODAS does not do the diagnosing; *You do!* In collaboration with your client, you can explore the answers and the implications of what those answers mean. For example, a client who is seen in your office on a weekly basis, might answer questions in the participation domain that give a clue to his or her isolation or opportunities to engage in healthy, supportive activities. You might be providing excellent support and

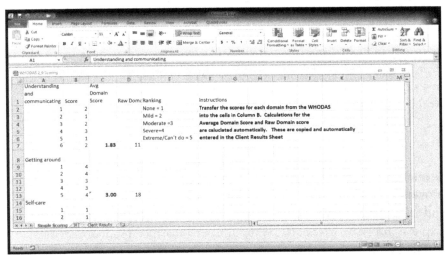

WHODAS Results: Excel Spreadsheet

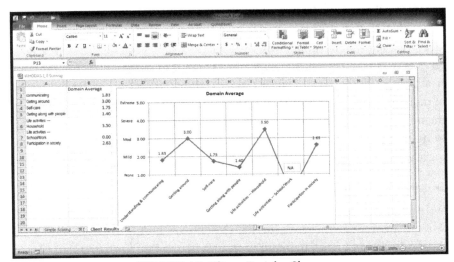

WHODAS Client Results Sheet

psychoeducation using CBT, but because your client lives in an area that has lots of barriers and they experience stigma at home for coming to see you, the progress they are making isn't what you had hoped. This instrument gives you an opportunity to explore these challenges in a manner that takes into account the responses (feelings, beliefs, experiences) of your clients such that you may address them from a more empathic stance.

I would encourage clinicians to use the WHODAS as a platform to explore your clients' strengths as well as discussing the barriers to successful treatment. Many of us find ways to adapt to changing situations. Our clients may have to utilize more energy to address these changes because of the barriers they experience. Our professional skill sets lend themselves to brainstorming and exploring functionality that our clients may have overlooked, dismissed, or never accessed. Providing opportunities to practice new skills in a supportive, therapeutic environment is key to generalizing these to 'real-world' experiences.

USING THE INFORMATION WITH OTHER PROFESSIONALS

Assuming a collaborative stance with other treatment professionals is key to providing our clients with ethical and sustainable treatment. A well-recognized and validated instrument such as the WHODAS 2.0 is like using an American Express card – you have entrée without having to explain source material. Depending on the scope of your practice and the focus of your work with your client, you may find using the WHODAS is useful in sharing your insights into your client's functioning with others such as primary care providers.

The WHODAS may provide useful information for advocating for services for clients. This can be in several different domains ranging from school services to disability evaluations. It can be useful in determining priorities for treatment planning. If your client cannot get to your office for services because of mobility, then the priority for treatment is finding a way to bring treatment to them. If your client cannot concentrate, focus on a conversation, or remember to do things, then these must be addressed as part of the work you are doing together.

Treatment planning and the WHODAS 2.0

Writing a treatment plan using WHODAS 2.0 results is fairly straightforward. You can incorporate the results domain by domain, and/or you can summarize the results giving a general disability score. This is a far more psychometrically sound method of evaluating global assessment of functioning than the GAF.

Examples of how the WHODAS was incorporated into treatment plans for different ages and situations follow. The identities of the clients used in these case studies have been changed to protect confidentiality, but accurately reflect the issues presented in treatment and the use of the WHODAS in identifying, tracking, and fostering change.

CASE STUDY 1: SALLY

Sally was referred to me by her neurologist. Sally was 45 years-old and divorced. She was on disability and lived in subsidized housing. Her presenting issues were depression, anxiety, and difficulty with pain management. Sally had a very creative and entrepreneurial spirit. She had a difficult childhood that included physical and emotional abuse, but she found connection with one of her teachers in high school who encouraged her. Once she graduated from high school, she moved out of her family home. She hung with other young adults, smoked weed, drank, and eventually ended up becoming pregnant by one of her "friends." She elected to have the baby and actually blossomed when she took on the responsibility of raising her daughter. She received support from various social service agencies and continued on to get an associate degree from the local community college. She was able to support herself and her daughter through working several jobs, and made amends with her mother who watched the baby. She was doing well and making ends meet when she was in a car accident that left her with head, neck, and back injuries. These injuries resolved, but left her with mild cognitive deficits and chronic pain issues. By the time I saw her, she had effectively been under-employed for over 20 years, had developed dependency on a variety of pain medications, and was quite dependent financially on supplemental security disability income (SSDI). She augmented these funds with making and selling jewelry online. Her daughter was her caregiver, and the two of them lived in supported housing. She drove, but only occasionally, as she was uncomfortable both physically and psychologically. Most of the time she spent in her apartment, but connected with others through social media and Skype.

I gave Sally the 36-question, self-administered WHODAS 2.0. Sally's Global Disability Score was 134 out of a possible 180. She believed that this accurately reflected her experience during the previous 30-day period. She had endorsed lower levels of disability in the domains of understanding and communicating with others, and had endorsed maximum levels of disability in life activities (household and work), and near maximum in participation in society.

Further conversations, however, suggested that while she could not work and had difficulty taking care of the house, she did not feel any limitation in this regard, because her daughter was there to support her. We agreed, however, that if her daughter were to leave, these areas would become a focus of her anxiety and stress. Her strengths in communicating became crucial in addressing her vulnerabilities. So one aspect of our treatment became skills-building in assertiveness and negotiating successfully with others to make sure her needs were met.

Subsequent administrations of the WHODAS revealed positive changes in her ability to get around and care for herself as her pain management skills improved. We worked together with her neurologist to monitor and modify her pain medication protocols and confirmed these changes with the monthly self-reports she provided the neurologist which became very useful for Sally's quarterly visits.

Sally felt empowered to address some elements that she had previously given up hope for changing. Her cognition improved as she became more willing to go out of her apartment and engaged more in fun activities, rather than just going to doctors' appointments. She began to advocate for herself and others in similar situations. The feedback from these activities encouraged her to start an exercise program that her neurologist had been recommending for some time. All of these efforts resulted in gains for Sally and she was able to capture these changes on the WHODAS.

CASE STUDY 2: AIDAN AND HIS MOM, EMILY

Aidan was a 15 year-old who came from a mixed-race, divorced family. His mother, Emily, was a recovering meth addict. Her children had been taken from her while she was actively using meth by Child Protective Services. She had successfully undergone treatment and was now in the process of reunification. Aidan, her middle child, was quite rebellious, and she was seeking help for him so that he wouldn't end up like she did. Aidan was brought to therapy against his will. He didn't think he had any problems, and wasn't interested in talking to anybody about anything. The 12-question version of the WHODAS covers all six domains, but adds an element of evaluation specifically asking the person to summarize how many days during the past 30 they experienced the problems, were totally unable to carry out usual activities, and/or had to cut back or reduce activities because of the health condition. I chose to the use the 12-question version with Aidan because I didn't think he would cooperate and complete the full 36-question version, and I used the proxy with his mother to make sure I calibrated their responses.

Aidan had already been evaluated in school and was found to have attention deficit/hyper activity disorder. He had been asked to leave both his public school and the continuation school because of his behaviors and because of his use of substances. Emily wanted me to work with Aidan to address his anger and his substance use.

Aidan, as might be expected, didn't think he had problems with much of anything, but it was interesting that for the two items he did identify (concentrating for 10 minutes and dealing with people he did not know), he indicated he had problems for 20 days out of the 30. This became my entry point with him. I inquired about what was getting in the way of his being able to concentrate and how that interfered with his goals, and followed-up on his inability to deal with people he did not know by asking him how it would be to work with someone like me.

His mother's evaluation of her son was quite different, with Emily endorsing "extreme" or "severe" on 8 out of 12 items. I was able to use this in working with Aidan to ask him why others might see his behaviors differently from himself and began a conversation about how he felt judged and how this got him to behave in ways he was not happy with. I reinforced Emily's positive parenting skills, noting that she was obviously concerned enough about Aidan's functioning to seek out support.

The WHODAS allowed me to enter into this family system as a neutral (or nearly neutral) third party rather than as an enforcer. We used the WHODAS to monitor changes. Emily's proxy came down in intensity, and Aidan's became more self-honest.

CASE STUDY 3: ALICE, A RESIDENT IN
AN ASSISTED LIVING FACILITY

Alice was 84 when I first met her. She was referred to me by her primary care physician who was helping her get through a bout of shingles. The pain had triggered a debilitating anxiety response which was making treatment problematic. I worked with Alice for over two years, and as our therapeutic relationship developed, the answers to the WHODAS evolved.

Alice played many roles in her lifetime—wife, mother, educator, administrator, but in her heart she was always an artist. When she was in her 30's, her husband died unexpectedly, and Alice needed to get a job to support the family. She found work fairly easily, as she was college-educated, and had skills. While this was difficult for her children, it was a necessary adjustment that the whole family made. Her children left home, began lives of their own, and Alice continued in her career. She never remarried. By the time she retired, she had accumulated a lovely nest egg and decided that she would insure her future care by buying into a graduated living situation where she could move from independent living to assisted living to full care, if needed. She thoroughly involved herself in this community, acted as a board member, participated in the many activities provided to residents, and made supportive, lasting friendships.

She had positive, if occasionally rocky, relationships with her children and seemed to be enjoying life fully until her physical body began to fail her. She experienced decline in her activities of daily living, began to withdraw from the offerings of the site, and began to re-experience a deep depression with associated anxiety that had actually been life-long. The pain exacerbated her experiences, and she was put on a variety of medications (anti-depressants and anxiolytics) that frustrated her because they did little to alleviate her physical and emotional pain, but made her realize that she was no longer the strong, independent woman she had always been.

While she was cognitively intact, I decided to use the WHODAS 2.0 12+24 interview because it gave me a way to ask questions that might have been experienced as intrusive if not in this interview format. The interview is scripted and focuses on "health conditions", a term that avoids the stigma of identifying a "mental illness", but screens for it all the same. This is particularly useful for this generation, as there is a negative perception about having mental illness that sometimes precludes the individual's seeking help. The 12+24 is also interactive, in that it provides flashcards for the interviewee to use in forming their responses.

This version is divided into core questions and continuation questions. If the core questions are endorsed with a rating of "none", then the interview is ended. If, on the other hand, any of the core questions is endorsed with "mild", "moderate", "severe", or "extreme", then the continuation questions are asked. Based on the answers to the continuation questions, specific domains of functioning are then explored. This tiered interview allows the interviewer to follow up on specific domains of functioning that are problematic without having to ask all 36 questions.

Alice was initially interviewed when she was in the skilled nursing unit at the site. She was in a great deal of pain, and didn't have capacity or tolerance for a long interview. She endorsed problems in four out of the five core questions, identifying severity levels of "severe" or "extreme" for these. The seven continuation questions elicited responses in five, with severity levels of "mild", "moderate", and "severe". Based on these answers, I drilled down into the domains of mobility, self, care, life activities, and self-care. The interview took approximately 15 minutes.

I had accumulated a great deal of information from this one interview, and it was not unduly taxing to my client. After she was discharged from the SNF and returned to her apartment, we continued to use the WHODAS to monitor her change as she recovered and implemented the mindfulness and stress reduction skills we went over in treatment. Since this was a long-term therapeutic relationship, we revisited several of the items over time to see how things had changed. This provided a very useful picture of her overall functioning, which she shared with her primary care provider who, in turn, was able to better address her pain issues.

WHODAS PILOT IN AN AGENCY

I asked colleagues to pilot the WHODAS in an agency setting to see what some of the challenges might be. The agency (Social Advocates for Youth) offers crisis, counseling, and community programs throughout Sonoma County in Northern California. They serve diverse at-risk and high-needs populations through age 25, including children who have been physically, sexually or emotionally abused or who are at risk of abuse, runaway and homeless youth, transitional age youth (former foster youth and homeless young adults), youth at risk of gang involvement, young parents, youth seeking guidance in finding jobs and completing their education, and youth who may be struggling in their transition from teen to young adulthood.

Clinicians generally found the information obtained useful in providing treatment to their clients. They found value in using it to monitor change, especially in cases where there was chronicity of disability arising from situational factors (e.g., poverty, transportation, etc.). One participant noted that the clients had not considered aspects of their situation as being disability-related. In looking at it this way, the clients felt validated in that their experiences were taken into account, not just their diagnoses. Clinicians also felt the WHODAS was useful in starting conversations about broader topics than behavioral issues. These conversations allowed for a deeper therapeutic rapport to be developed. More information on this pilot can be found in Chapter 7.

There were some challenges with the measure. Clinicians did note that without sufficient orientation to the WHODAS, administration and scoring were confusing. I have made attempts to address these concerns in Chapter 7.

CONCLUSION

As this chapter has shown, there are multiple uses for the WHODAS with clients of different ages and different issues those clients may have. The instrument itself doesn't diagnose, rather it provides clinicians with opportunities to engage with and explore issues that their clients are facing. It also monitors where changes are occurring during the relationship. Where these changes are positive, it is possible to reinforce the gains and expand the learning and application to other domains. Where changes are negative, it is useful for identifying opportunities, relapse prevention, advocacy, and to monitor for shifting priorities in treatment.

The three versions provided allow for clinicians to determine which best meets the abilities of the client and the needs of the clinician. Since the instrument has been well-tested throughout the world in many different settings, clinicians can rely on the reliability of the responses and know that the questions actually elicit information that is valuable in identifying treatment goals and measuring outcomes.

CHAPTER 3

Symptom Severity Measures

INTRODUCTION

A challenge faced by every clinician is identifying what actually is happening for our client(s). Information gathered at intake may reveal some of what is going on, but not necessarily everything that is occurring. One way we have to minimize overlooking something important is to systematically explore all domains of functioning.

I was trained by a psychologist who had done his post-doc at the Menninger Clinic. His training was rigorous, and he made sure that my training was equally rigorous. The patient history I was trained on was seven pages long and included detailed exploration of gestational, developmental, psychosocial, educational, and psychological aspects of the individual. Using this model was challenging, especially with patients who were low functioning, not only because it took so long, but also because there were frequent gaps in knowledge because the patient was unwilling or unable to share it. While I appreciate this model in terms of learning how to do a thorough history, it takes an enormous amount of time to gather, and at times feels intrusive. And while it is important to assess each of the areas, I always felt there had to be a more efficient or productive way to obtain this information.

Gathering an adequate history sufficient to identify the presenting issue and develop a treatment plan takes time, and requires frequent revision. Not all therapeutic situations lend themselves to this process. One of the tools provided in the DSM-5 to address this challenge is the awkwardly entitled, "Level 1 Cross-Cutting Symptom Measures".

According to the DSM-5 website (http://www.psychiatry.org/practice/dsm/dsm5/onlineassessment-measures):

- Cross-cutting symptom measures may aid in a comprehensive mental status assessment by drawing attention to symptoms that are important across diagnoses. They are intended to help identify additional areas of inquiry that may guide treatment and prognosis. The cross-cutting measures have two levels: Level 1 questions are a brief survey of 13 domains for adult patients and 12 domains for child and adolescent patients, and Level 2 questions provide a more in-depth assessment of certain domains.

- Severity measures are disorder-specific, corresponding closely to criteria that constitute the disorder definition. They may be administered to individuals who have received a diagnosis or who have a clinically significant syndrome that falls short of meeting full criteria. Some of the assessments are self-completed, whereas others require a clinician to complete.

Some readers will be familiar with the Symptom Checklist-90-Revised. While not acknowledged in the DSM-5, it could be inferred that this was the model for development of the Cross-Cutting Symptom Measures. Rationale for including this approach lies in recognition that most psychological disorders are not neatly categorized, but are more heterogeneous, with symptoms appearing across a spectrum of behaviors, beliefs, and cognitions. This is consistent with the dimensional evaluation basis of the DSM-5. Having an assessment that explores symptoms across domains of functioning will provide the clinician with a more dimensional view of the client. Clinicians can then construct with the client a treatment plan that addresses more than just symptoms.

Domains of Functioning

The domains of functioning identified in the Level 1 are: somatic symptoms, sleep problems, inattention, depression, anger, irritability, mania, anxiety, psychosis, repetitive thoughts and behaviors, substance use and suicidal idea/or attempts. Once areas of problematic functioning are identified, there are follow-up assessments (Level-2) for each domain that can be used to track change.

These assessments, in and of themselves, are not diagnostic. The Level-1 and Level-2 measures are useful in exploring symptoms in depth and addressing the areas where providers can collaborate. They are useful for identifying areas for treatment and measuring change.

These measures are also useful in working with individuals who have complex presentations. For example, it is not uncommon for clients to experience problems with sleep, substance use, anger, and depression. Clinicians may collaborate in the continuum of care with other providers such as primary care physicians or nurse practitioners, substance abuse counselors, and psychiatrists who are addressing more specialized aspects of the client's overall functioning. Using the Level-1 and Level-2 measures, information can be shared across specialties and assessment of all domains of functioning monitored using one instrument.

The balance of this chapter will look at how the Level-1 was developed, discuss the measures in depth, discuss scoring and interpretation, and then provide case examples for implementing this in a private practice or agency or group setting.

DEVELOPMENT

The Patient-Reported Outcomes Measurement Information System (PROMIS) represents work started in 2004 by a group of outcomes scientists from seven institutions and the National Institutes of Health (NIH). The initiatives funded by NIH were designed to transform medical research capabilities and share discoveries with practitioners. These initiatives also sought to be useful and were not just published for researchers. (Anonymous, NIH, 2009). If you are interested in the development of these, more information on the process can be found at http://www.nihpromis.org.

The American Psychiatric Association participated in this initiative during its revision of the DSM, and the combined efforts produced 12 new tools for use by clinicians in evaluating and further exploring symptoms in young children, adolescents, and adults. These tools have passed rigorous psychometric testing and are both valid and reliable. They are found on the DSM-5 website (www.DSM5.org) and can be downloaded and copied without restriction for clinical use.

Additional measures were identified from existing assessments and modified to meet the needs of the DSM-5. These instruments include the widely used Patient Health Questionnaire (PHQ-9), National Institute on Drug Abuse's Alcohol, Smoking and Substance Involvement Screening Test (NIDA-Modified ASSIST), Children's Florida Obsessive Compulsive Inventory [C-FOCI] Severity Scale, Altman Self-Rating Mania Scale [ASRM]), Affective Reactivity Index [ARI]), Swanson, Nolan, and Pelham, version IV [SNAP-IV]), National Stressful Events Survey Acute Stress Disorder Short Scale [NSESS]), Brief Dissociative Experiences Scale [DES-B]); DES-B modified for DSM-5 (Dalenberg & Carlson 2010).

Description of the Level 1 Cross-Cutting Symptoms for Adults

This screen consists of 23 questions that cover 13 domains of functioning. The domains are: depression, anger, mania, anxiety, somatization, suicidal ideation, psychosis, sleep problems, memory, repetitive thoughts and behaviors, dissociation, personality functioning, and substance use. Each domain is covered by one to three questions. Each of the questions is answered based on the individual's experience (how much they have been "bothered by" a particular symptom) during the past two weeks. Responses include "none" (not at all), "slight" (rare, less than a day or two), "mild" (several days), "moderate" (more than half the days), and "severe" (nearly every day). The form uses Roman numerals and shading to demark the various domains rather than listing them. For example, Roman numeral I consists of two questions to screen for depression and Roman numeral XIII has three questions to screen for substance use.

Versions of the Level-1 form for children (ages 6-11), adolescents (ages 11-17) and adults (ages 18 and up) can be downloaded from the DSM-5 website (www.dsm5.org). Hard copy versions of the adult and parent/guardian versions for children can be found in the back of the DSM-5 full-edition, in Section III, but not the pocket edition.

Description of the Level 1 Cross-Cutting Symptoms for Parent/Guardian for Children 6-17

This screen is organized a bit differently from the adult version. It contains 25 questions covering 12 domains. These domains, while substantively the same as for the adult, do have some evaluative differences. The domains are: somatic symptoms, sleep problems, inattention, depression, anger, irritability, mania, anxiety, psychosis, repetitive thoughts and behaviors, substance use and suicidal ideation/attempts. Parents or guardians are asked to respond on the same 5-point Likert scale of "none", "slight", "mild", "moderate", and "severe" rating concerns with behavior over the past two weeks. The substance use domain is the only one scored on a "yes/no or don't know" basis. As with the adult screen results, clinicians should follow up on any endorsement of "mild" or higher.

Each domain is covered by one to four questions. As with the adult version, the form uses Roman numerals and shading to demark the various domains rather than listing them. For example, Roman numeral I consists of two questions to screen for somatic symptoms and Roman numeral III has one question to screen for inattention. Substance use and suicidal ideation/attempts are screened using six questions with "yes", "no", or "don't know" responses.

Description of the Level 2 Screens

There are over 50 additional screens that can be used for follow-up. They are found on the DSM-5 website and are grouped into age- (self-report) and disorder-specific severity sets (clinician-administered). These can be given to clients who already have a diagnosis or who have symptoms that fall short of meeting full criteria for a particular diagnosis. The reader will find a table that identifies each of the screens by name, age group, type of administration (self, proxy, or clinician), scoring protocol, and source in Appendix D.

The screens are very brief and would be useful for monitoring, but do not provide much in the way of additional information for diagnostic purposes. They are also useful as teaching tools for students and/or interns, as they are primarily symptom-specific and relate directly to the descriptions in the DSM-5 for the various disorders. They may be useful for some clients in educating them about their symptoms and helping them to more accurately track them.

APPLICATIONS

Practitioners will find it useful to provide the Level-1 screen to new clients. Because it is a systematic survey of behavioral functioning, it can both help to gather information and supplement information identified in the intake or first session.

A useful metaphor here may be thinking of the Level-1 screen as a triage tool. The DSM-5 recommends that individuals who respond with scores that are at or above the threshold "mild", would benefit from further evaluation in those areas. Your client's endorsement of higher levels of impairment may depend on the issue that brought him or her in. It also may reflect his/her level of denial or readiness for change. Using the screen to help focus the treatment can be an effective way to enter into the therapeutic relationship and insure that the client's needs are being met.

It stands to reason that successful interventions should result in a decrease in intensity of symptoms and, the Level-1 screen, when used as a follow-up tool, will typically reflect that. Where it does not, the clinician then has an opportunity to evaluate the client's ability to benefit from the intervention, to change the intervention, and adjust the treatment plan.

USING THIS INFORMATION WITH CLIENTS

"Does this mean I'm crazy?" Whether this question is explicit or implicit, people want to know what results mean. We want to believe that by answering some questions we can find the "hidden truth." Unlike the questionnaires found on "Dr. Google", the Level-1 screen is more of a shopping list than an archeological dig. How you share the results with your client is very important. Most importantly, however, is *that* you share the results with them.

We are living in an age where information can be readily and easily downloaded and shared. Many Millennials and Boomers are using apps on their Smart Phones to monitor health outcomes. Because there is an expectation for information to be provided in visual form, I share responses to these questionnaires with my clients visually. This provides shared ownership of the results, as well as defusing some of the stigma and misunderstanding around words such as "psychosis" and "suicidal ideation". It also goes a long way in challenging the belief that somehow, as a psychologist, I can read minds!

I created a report that I share with my clients. You can find a copy in the Forms section. Producing the report requires several steps. You need to enter the scores into an Excel spreadsheet, cut and paste the chart created into the report document, then provide an interpretation of what the scores mean. This last step requires that you apply your clinical expertise to the information and infer and interpret the scores. There are no canned answers here! Each time you use the Level-1, you would need to re-create the report.

This approach reflects my ignorance of how to develop an app, and my own preference how to put a report together. I am certain that there are more efficient and effective ways to share this information. I know that there are individuals who will be reading this who can and will develop something. My hope is that this can be shared with all clinicians!

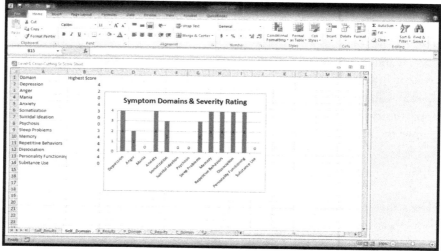

Level 1: Adult (Self) Score

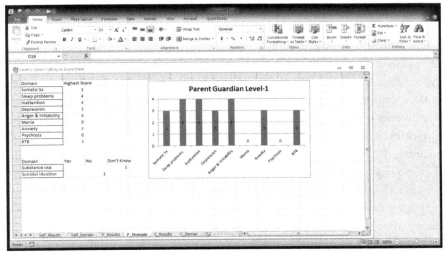

Level 1: Parent Results

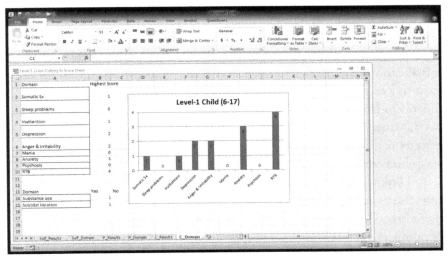

Level 1: Child

ADMINISTRATION AND SCORING OF LEVEL 1 SCREEN

Instructions on how to score the results are included in each instrument. Basically, this is a self-report using a 5-point Likert scale. Higher scores indicate greater severity. As noted above, the domains covered in the instrument are depression, anger, mania, anxiety, somatic symptoms, suicidal ideation, psychosis, sleep problems, memory, repetitive thoughts and behaviors, dissociation, personality functioning, and substance use. Any domain scored at 2 or higher (a fairly low threshold), should be investigated further. Because of the variability of mood and developmental stages, frequent administration of this screen can be particularly useful.

There are several considerations in scoring the Level-1 Parent/Guardian version. Clinicians are directed to pay attention to the score on each item within a domain and then note the highest score in the column provided. This works until you get to the substance use and suicidal ideation/attempt questions. There are no weights assigned to the "yes", "no", or "don't know" answers. The instructions provide a table with a "threshold guide for further inquiry", which recommends follow-up with "don't know" answers. This suggests that the "don't know" is of more concern than the "yes". Clinicians may agree or disagree with this, but I suggest that responses of "yes" and "don't know" should be considered red flags and acted on accordingly.

Interpretation and Use

Scoring the instrument is just the jumping-off place. In my experience, few of my clients actually have a single-issue presentation. Most have flavors of anxiety and depression, as well as substance use and sleep problems. It would be a mistake to use the Level-1 solely to document problems when it can be used to further explore how your client(s) has/have negotiated their lives with these functional issues present. This is where the Cultural Formulation Interview (see Chapter 5) and the WHODAS 2.0 (see Chapter 2) can be integrated to get a more dimensional view of your client's functioning and his or her capacity to function, given their current circumstances.

Looking at raw data from these instruments is similar to reading results from your blood tests. Unless you know what is being measured, what the "normal" range of response is, and what the outliers are, it's just a bunch of numbers. So it is important that *before* using the instrument, you look at how and what things are being measured. Any scores of mild, moderate, or severe should be used to address specific issues within the treatment plan. Keep in mind that functional impairment is not just about "how many" symptoms a person endorses. That person may be able to function in spite of their challenges. The implication that more symptoms at higher degrees of severity equates with impairment needs to be explored individually.

Frequency of Administration

Frequency of administration depends on how well the client is functioning and how severe the symptoms are. If symptoms are found to be "none", "slight", or "mild", you might use the instrument as a follow-up at discharge. If the symptoms are "moderate" or "severe", you might use the instrument more frequently to monitor changes. Currently there are no explicit standards for frequency of administration. A rule of thumb that may be useful is for chronically ill clients (i.e., those with treatment-resistant diagnoses such as schizophrenia or personality disorders), you might choose to administer these once or twice a year. For individuals who have presentations that are episodic, you may choose to administer at intake, after the first five or six visits, and then at discharge.

Billing and Coding

Questions occasionally arise as to whether insurance companies will pay for administration and scoring time. What payers determine is reimbursable is their decision, and if you are on an insurance panel, you are subject to their conditions. Depending on your scope of practice, however, there are CPT codes that can be used for these purposes. The trend in coding, billing and documentation of services is toward monitoring change. A case might be made that if you DO NOT include these measures, you may be at risk for being asked for repayment. Further, from a risk management stance, documentation of change may provide you with evidence that you were acting competently should you ever be challenged in a malpractice suit.

Self-Report Measures and Clinical Judgment

Remember that these are self-report measures. It is vital that the clients understand that *their assessment of what is going on for them* is what is being measured. Will some clients exaggerate their symptoms? Yes, of course. Will others underplay their symptoms? Yes, of course. The screens are not lie-detectors. They are just one aspect of using clinical judgment to arrive at a treatment hypothesis. They are an efficient way of gathering information consistently over time. It is like having a shopping list to remind you to look for things you need.

USING THIS INFORMATION WITH OTHER PROFESSIONALS

HIPAA Issues and Confidentiality

It is important to note that HIPAA was designed to improve communication between providers, not hinder it. Obtaining releases of information for sharing of these types of assessments is encouraged, but more importantly, working with your client(s) to empower him/her/them to actively participate in the evaluation process and share that information with all their care providers is paramount. Raw data should not be handed out without making sure that the information is understandable. Typically this is done by providing a summary of the results and a description of the implications.

The summary of the results should include a statement about the instrument and a brief description of what it is designed to do. Results can be summarized in terms of areas that need attention, areas needing improvement, outliers, and norms (if relevant). Examples of these summaries are found in the case studies at the end of this chapter.

When sharing this information with other care providers, such as primary care physicians, it is helpful to add a statement of how you are using the results with your clients. For example, if you are working with someone who is depressed, it is useful to also include information on other related symptoms that were endorsed so that the physician is alerted to other possible underlying physiological issues.

Clustering

You will want to explore domains that are endorsed at "mild" or higher. These may show up in clusters. For example, depression, anxiety, and somatic symptoms may cluster together. When you add a "moderate" or "severe" endorsement for suicidal ideation to this cluster, you can more accurately predict risk and make a strong case for additional support or need for services.

Similarly, when you note a reduction in levels of endorsement, you can reasonably expect other domains to see reductions. If this is not happening, you may explore this with the client to determine if there are contributory issues that need to be addressed by other professionals. For example, if there is a reduction in anxiety and suicidal ideation, but not depression, you may want to refer your client to a nutritionist, endocrinologist, or neurologist to rule out food allergies, diabetes, or Parkinson's.

Level-2 Measures

As noted above, there are over 50 additional measures to use as follow-up with symptom-specific evaluation. In looking through these and in piloting them in my own practice, I did not find much diagnostic utility. I did, however, find them useful for educating my clients about their symptoms and explaining how I came to my diagnosis. This proved valuable for those clients who were more pro-active about their illness. For others, the information did not prove to be enlightening.

Readers who are involved with training interns might find the Level-2 measures useful for better understanding various symptoms found within a given diagnostic category. Readers who are involved in program evaluation and outcomes studies will find these shorter measures useful as monitors for assessing change.

CASE STUDY 1: ARNIE

Arnie is a 57 year-old teacher, father, and self-described "workaholic". He is very active and involved in lots of different things. He and his wife have been married for 37 years. Arnie came to see me because he was concerned about his memory. He had gotten a clean bill of health from his primary care physician, wasn't on any medications, and on the surface, appeared to be experiencing challenges with a life transition. He shared that there had been a lot of stress in his jobs, and related that his daughter had lost her husband in a traumatic accident recently. He also noted that his wife had problems with her mother who was getting older and needing more support. He assured me that he really loved what he was doing for his work, but admitted that he didn't always know how to say "No" and was feeling pulled in many different directions. He also shared that he was quite worried about his wife and daughter.

On the surface, this appeared to be fairly classic adjustment disorder. I asked Arnie to complete the Level-1 and his responses shocked me. I shared the following chart with him to begin our conversation about what concerned him most.

10 of the 13 domains were endorsed with at least one question at a severity level of moderate or severe. This indicated far more stress than what Arnie had led me to believe. We began our work with acknowledging that

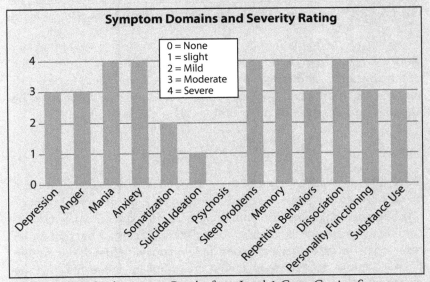

Chart 1 Case Study: Arnie – Results from Level-1 Cross-Cutting Symptom Measure with Severity

Arnie was feeling very overwhelmed emotionally. Together we decided that there were some things he could change immediately that might decrease the levels of severity (e.g., getting more exercise and doing pleasurable activities, renegotiating deadlines and commitments). This gave him a sense of ownership in the process and a measurable goal to work with.

I saw Arnie on a weekly basis for our first several visits. After two months of work together using a combination of CBT and mindfulness-based stress reduction, Arnie completed the Level-1 a second time. His results are below.

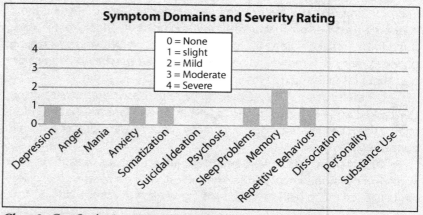

Chart 2 Case Study: Arnie – Level-1 Cross Cutting Symptom Measure at two months

This was a dramatic shift that was confirmation to Arnie that our work was resulting in changes. He admitted that he hadn't thought much of therapy before, and really wondered whether it was going to be worth his time. Using the Level-1 screen helped him to see that the changes he was making were showing up in lots of ways in his life.

CASE STUDY 2: SONIA

Sonia, a 17- year old girl, came to me at the request of her stepmother who was concerned that Sonia was not performing up to her potential in school. She had been doing well up until her last year in high school, when, according to her stepmother, she "suddenly" started to ignore her homework resulting in her grades falling, began hanging out with friends her mother did not approve of, and was no longer the compliant, agreeable child she had been up until this point. There was a history of depression in the family, and there were stressors including a blended family, economic issues, and a history of early loss. Sonia's birth mother had died in a car accident when Sonia was just 4 years-old. She had been raised by her maternal grandmother until she turned 16 when she was re-united with her birth father and his wife.

Sonia's stepmother was genuinely concerned for her daughter, and wanted to make sure that Sonia had opportunities to discuss her feelings about all that had happened to her in her short life. Sonia was willing to see me. In order to establish some therapeutic alliance, my first visit with Sonia consisted of our discussing whether she agreed with her stepmother's concerns. I shared the following results with her (with her stepmother's permission). The Level-1 Parent-Guardian Screen was used.

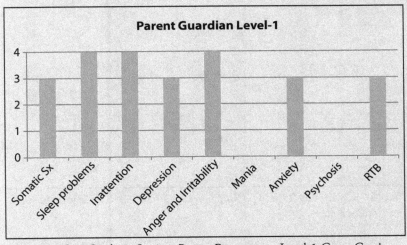

Chart 3   Case Study 2: Sonia – Parent Response to Level-1 Cross-Cutting Symptom Measure

Sonia's response as we looked over the chart was fascinating. She was quite engaged with the notion that her behaviors could be looked at in this light, and she agreed that there was some accuracy in how her step-mother had scored her in these domains. I then gave Sonia the child version of the Level-1 and asked her to fill it out with the understanding that we would explore her perceptions and see where there were differences and where there were similarities. Her results are shown on next page.

As may be expected, Sonia's responses were less severe than her stepmother's, but there were congruencies in the domains. I suggested to Sonia that this might reflect her concerns about her future or it might reflect issues from her past. I expressed my concern about her responses to specific items endorsed that resulted in high domain scores—specifically, one on having thought about something bad happening to her or someone else. We used this to do some work on her mother's death. I used the incongruences in endorsement on use of substances (Sonia endorsed "yes", Step-mom endorsed "Don't Know") as an opportunity to provide some psychoeducation and explore with Sonia why she was experimenting with drugs and alcohol.

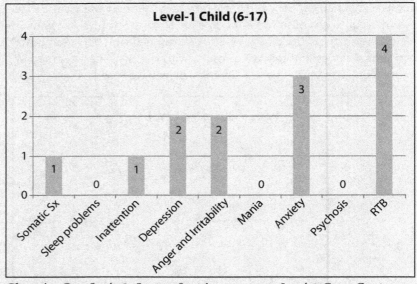

Chart 4 Case Study 2: Sonia – Sonia's responses to Level-1 Cross-Cutting Symptom Measure

The most enlightening response, however, was Sonia's endorsement of having attempted suicide. This was not something she had ever shared with her step-mom. We used several sessions to explore her experience and how she had decided she would be better off dead, as well as to address her underlying depression and anxiety. Sonia felt she had worked through the problem after several sessions and decided she was ready to move on. My conclusion was that without the screen, she might never have shared her suicide attempt with an adult. The screen allowed the conversation to begin.

CONCLUSION

The Level-1 Cross Cutting Symptom Measure is a very useful instrument that captures lots of information in a relatively easy-to-use format. Different versions of the measure allow clinicians to gather information different ways.

It is also very useful in measuring changes over time. Drawbacks include lack of translations in languages other than English.

While there are an overwhelming number of Level-2 measures, it may be useful to explore using them with clients both as a means of measuring symptom-specific changes and as a way of educating clients about their symptoms. Additionally, these measures are useful for training students and interns as they capture essential symptomatology on a brief form.

Finally, these measures provide a way to monitor effectiveness of interventions and changes in intensity of symptoms. Periodic administration is straightforward, and results may provide clients with more ownership of their treatment. When used in agency or group settings, these measures can be used to monitor outcomes, as well as to train staff.

Scoring and charts for the Level-1 Cross-Cutting Symptoms can be found in Form A at the back of the book.

CHAPTER 4

Clinician-Rated Measures

The measures discussed in the previous chapters have all been self-report measures. This chapter will discuss six clinician-rated instruments developed by the DSM-5 authors that can be used to evaluate behaviors found across different disorders. These measures, as with the others found on the DSM-5 website, are in the public domain and can be used for clinical purposes without violating any copyright laws. They can be used to monitor changes in frequency and duration of specific symptoms, or changes in behavior. They may also be useful for monitoring changes when medications are introduced or changed.

As a psychologist, part of my basic training and ongoing professional development was in psychological assessment. It is useful to remember that training in administering, scoring, and interpreting psychological tests and measures is NOT typically part of medical education, and only a small part of training in most master's level psychology programs. At first glance, it may appear that it is easy to administer and score the clinician-rated measures contained in the DSM-5, but I would challenge that assumption and encourage all clinicians to follow the applicable ethical guidelines regarding limitations in administering or interpreting tests and measures that they may be subject to.

Going to the DSM5.org website and clicking the link for Online Assessment Measures under "What's New" and scrolling approximately two-thirds of the way down will bring you to six clinician-rated instruments. These are diagnostically useful, brief rating scales specific to several disorders: oppositional defiant disorder, conduct disorder, autism spectrum and social communication disorders, psychosis symptom severity (also available in print book), somatic symptom disorder, and non-suicidal self-injury. Each instrument contains instructions on scoring and frequency of use. They do not include interpretation of results.

SCORING AND INTERPRETATION

With minor variations within a specific instrument, all these are scored on a 5-point Likert scale, with the clinician exercising clinical judgment in assigning levels of severity. Unlike the client self-report measures, there is no weighting of individual questions or summing of domains to determine overall severity. Each item should be viewed as separate and distinct, and used for designing specific interventions when treatment planning.

One of the challenges in using clinician-rated scales is that without some training to insure inter-rater reliability, one person's "extreme" is another's "mild". To address this variability, the DSM-5 provides thumbnail descriptors for each of the Likert-points. Even with that, however, these measures are subject to great variability in assignment of rankings. Psychologists recognize this and will typically use several measures to identify and explore issues. There is no such recommendation in the DSM-5, which is a threat to the overall utility of this information. As a provider, it would be prudent to make sure you are evaluating not just the symptoms, but the overall functioning of your client. Thus you may want to refer the client to a psychologist for additional testing or, at a minimum, include several measures (self-report and clinician-rated) to improve the validity of the information.

The dilemma here lies more with inter-rater reliability than test-retest issues. If the measure is used as an inpatient monitor, it is essential that all clinicians who will be using it are trained on how to assess and evaluate patients using this measure. There may be more problems with outpatient evaluation as there is no specific training, and the evaluations will differ based on the clinician's level of training and experience with the disorder. As noted above, while the measures provide clear descriptions of the behaviors, there still is room for variability in evaluating severity. I believe we develop a type of clinical tolerance based on our backgrounds and clinical exposure to certain behaviors. What may be extreme behavior to a newly licensed clinician who has had little exposure to an individual experiencing a full-blown psychotic episode, may be "mild" or "moderate" to a clinician who has been practicing for several years in an in-patient setting. We need to remember that these are quantitative estimations of qualitative experiences.

FREQUENCY OF USE

A typical arc of use would include identifying the presence of the symptoms (baseline), and then following the course of the episode to assess reduction in or absence of symptoms over time. Since these measures are clinician-rated, there is no test-retest problem. In an outpatient setting, the clinician can use the measures on a weekly basis or less frequently. You may wish to do an initial evaluation (baseline), then follow up in several weeks. Or you may want to track specific symptoms for several weeks to see if there are any changes. In an inpatient setting, these measures can be used at each shift, daily, or weekly, depending on need and benefit.

Charting could be as simple as using the measure, filling in the boxes and putting the measure in the chart. The DSM-5 forms do not contain a space for the name of the clinician who is making the rating. This is an important oversight and should be addressed in your integration of these measures. If you are using an electronic health record (EHR), you can include these measures and the ratings within the program itself. There may be costs involved in uploading these and scoring them depending on which EHR you are using, so you should consult with the developer.

Measure Descriptions

The table below lists each of the measures. They are available at www.dsm5.org under "Online Assessment Measures".

Table 2 Clinician-Rated Severity Measures for specific disorders and conditions

Measure Name	Disorder	Age Group	Evaluation Period	Scoring	Source
Clinician-Rated Dimensions of Psychosis Symptom Severity	Psychosis	Child, adolescent, or adult	Past 7 days	8 domains of symptoms; 5-point Likert scale; scores **NOT** summed	American Psychiatric Association (also available in print book)
Clinician-Rated Severity of Somatic Symptom Disorder	Somatic Symptoms	Child, adolescent, or adult	Past 7 days	3-items; 5-point Likert scale; higher scores indicate severity	American Psychiatric Association

(Continued)

Table 2   (*Continued*)

Measure Name	Disorder	Age Group	Evaluation Period	Scoring	Source
Clinician-Rated Severity of Oppositional Defiant Disorder	Oppositional Defiant	Child, adolescent, or adult	Past 7 days	1 item; 4-point Likert Scale	American Psychiatric Association
Clinician-Rated Severity of Conduct Disorder	Conduct Disorder	Child, adolescent, or adult	Past 7 days	1 item; 4-point Likert Scale	American Psychiatric Association
Clinician-Rated Severity of Non-suicidal Self-Injury	Non-suicidal Self-injury	Child, adolescent, or adult	Past year	1 item; 4-point Likert Scale	American Psychiatric Association

The reader will note that most of these are one- or two-item measures. They ask the clinician to use all available information and clinical judgment to accurately select a level that is representative of the client's functioning for that particular item. Evaluation periods differ amongst the disorders ranging from the past 7 days to an entire year. Measures are completed at assessment. They are best used for treatment planning and prognosis, *not* diagnosis.

Each instrument looks at something a bit different and is noted in the table below.

Table 3   Specific Domains of Assessment in Clinician-Rated Measures

Area assessed	Assesses the . . .
Autism	level of interference in functioning and support required as a result of difficulties in 1) social communication and 2) restricted interests and repetitive behaviors that are present for the individual receiving care
Somatic Symptoms	severity of the individual's misattributions, excessive concerns, and/or preoccupations with the somatic symptom(s)
Oppositional Defiant	presence and severity of any oppositional defiant symptoms
Conduct Disorder	presence and severity of any conduct disorder symptoms
Non-suicidal Self-injury	presence and severity of any non-suicidal self-injury (NSSI) behaviors or problems

CLINICIAN-RATED DIMENSIONS OF PSYCHOSIS SYMPTOM SEVERITY SCALE

One of the philosophical and theoretical differences between the DSM-IV-TR and the DSM-5 is the idea of heterogeneity of disorders. In the DSM-5 world, psychosis appears in any number of different disorders (e.g., schizophrenia, bipolar disorder, substance use, delirium), and manifests itself differently in terms of severity and impairment in functional domains. The Clinician-Rated Dimensions of Psychosis Symptom Severity Scale is a useful tool to look at how psychosis manifests itself across diagnostic categories.

The instrument evaluates eight domains of functioning. These comprise positive symptoms (hallucinations, delusions, disorganized speech, and abnormal psychomotor behavior), negative behaviors, as well as impaired cognition, depression, and mania. Each of these domains is evaluated using a 5-point Likert scale, with specific examples of typical manifestations of the behaviors across the severity spectrum. Thus, you can evaluate the client's functioning over the past seven days looking at more than just whether a specific symptom is absent or present, and you can monitor overall functioning noting which domain(s) are more impacted. This allows clinicians to track the incredible variability of psychotic behavior in patients.

The scale goes from "0" (not present), "1" (equivocal), "2" (present but mild), "3" (present and moderate), and "4" (present and severe). These scales include descriptors for behaviors within each of the specific domains. For example, the descriptors for hallucinations (a positive symptom) include the following:

Table 4   Severity descriptions for Hallucinations in Clinician-Rated Psychosis Symptoms

0 Not present	1 Equivocal (severity or duration not sufficient to be considered psychosis)	2 Present, but mild, (little pressure to act upon voices, not very bothered by voices)	3 Present and moderate (some pressure to respond to voices, or is somewhat bothered by voices)	4 Present and severe (severe pressure to respond to voices, or is very bothered by voices)

Descriptors for negative symptoms are:

Table 5 Severity descriptions for Negative Symptoms in Clinician-Rated Psychosis Symptoms

0 Not present	1 Equivocal decrease in facial expressivity, prosody, gestures, or self-initiated behavior	2 Present, but mild, decrease in facial expressivity, prosody, gestures, or self-initiated behavior	3 Present and moderate decrease in facial expressivity, prosody, gestures, or self-initiated behavior	4 Present and severe decrease in facial expressivity, prosody, gestures, or self-initiated behavior

Reprinted with permission from the *Diagnostic and Statistical Manual of Mental Health Disorders*, Fifth Edition, (Copyright © 2013). American Psychiatric Association. All Rights Reserved.

Impaired cognition is evaluated according to standard deviations[1]

Table 6 Severity descriptions for Impaired Cognition in Clinician-Rated Psychosis Symptoms

0 Not present	1 Equivocal (cognitive function not clearly outside the range expected for age or SES; i.e., within 0.5 SD of mean)	2 Present, but mild, (some reduction in cognitive function; below expected for age and SES, 0.5–1 SD from mean)	3 Present and moderate (clear reduction in cognitive function; below expected for age and SES, 1–2 SD from mean)	4 Present and severe (severe reduction in cognitive function; below expected for age and SES, > 2 SD from mean)

Reprinted with permission from the *Diagnostic and Statistical Manual of Mental Health Disorders*, Fifth Edition, (Copyright © 2013). American Psychiatric Association. All Rights Reserved.

APPLICATIONS

The chart below shows data collected on a patient with schizoaffective disorder who was a resident of a skilled nursing facility. I tracked his symptoms over a six-week period during which time his medications were being adjusted. The adjustments were successful, and the scale captures the decrease in depression, negative behaviors, agitation, and hallucinations. This information was shared

---

[1] Here the standard deviation refers to the normal distribution of individuals. Thus, the mean is reflecting distribution of individuals with cognitive problems within the population. One standard deviation above or below the mean suggests that the client is already experiencing challenges, and should not be interpreted as "normal". As the standard deviations increase, the level of severity increases. Two standard deviations above the mean (if you recall from your statistics classes) represents the outer tail of the bell-shaped curve. This represents approximately 2.1% of the population and is, therefore, extreme or rare.

with his psychiatrist, who was able to follow the patient more closely. It also provided nursing home staff with information on specific issues related to the patient's interpersonal functioning that helped them in supporting the patient in engaging in healthier behaviors. No other clinician was rating this individual.

Data can be gathered over time and used to monitor changes in behavior and effectiveness of interventions.

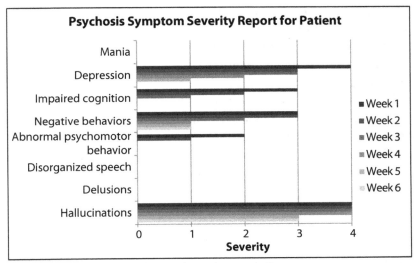

Chart 5   Sample Report for Psychosis Symptom Severity

Because the nursing staff saw improvement, I was asked to do an in-service training on psychosis in residents with mild and major neurocognitive disorders, personality disorders, and depression. This demonstrated to the facility staff that these behaviors occurred in a variety of organic disorders, not just "mental illness." Nurses were encouraged to use the scale to rate their patients and make referrals to behavioral health staff. Additional training was provided to the nursing staff in order to improve inter-rater reliability. The measure was uploaded to the EHR and the nursing staff would enter their rating along with other vital signs.

SHARING WITH CLIENTS

Historically, these types of data would have been summarized and shared with other professionals, but most likely not with the clients. My personal experience is that sometimes this information is useful to clients, and sometimes it is not. This invites clinicians to use our clinical judgment in sharing these results. You should also note, however, that the recent changes to the HIPAA law have expanded access to this type of information for clients. Depending on laws within your state, there may be additional rights extended to clients for obtaining this information.

Rather than state unequivocally that you should or should not provide this information, I would encourage you to consult with your local provider group, risk management (malpractice) providers, supervisors, and other similar resources to identify what is required in your specific locale. My personal practice is to share this information on a case-by-case basis in the interest of providing both information and insight to my clients. This may require my spending time explaining not just the results, but how they are determined and interpreting what these things mean. For the most part, this is usually not reimbursable.

This information may also be useful for other providers, especially primary care providers (e.g., physicians, nurse practitioners) who typically do not have a lot of time for narrative or explanation. Finding ways to succinctly state what the results show is important, and may be useful in the overall continuum of care for the client. It is important to reiterate that just sharing raw data with providers is not likely to be useful.

CONCLUSION

Clinician-rated scales are useful for monitoring specific symptoms over time. With proper training and collective understanding and agreement of what each of the descriptors means, clinicians can easily gather information and then use it to track the effectiveness of their interventions, adapt treatment plans, and chart overall changes in the client. These measures are vulnerable to several important areas of reliability. Inter-rater reliability may be low without sufficient training on the part of the individual who is making the rating and without sufficient training among individuals using the measure within an in-patient or group setting. Test-retest reliability is dependent on how well the staff have been trained to administer the measures.

Use of these monitors can extend from just keeping the ratings in the chart, to producing comparisons of changes over time. Incorporating this information and sharing it between providers is valuable. It may also be valuable to share this information with clients. This is an area for clinical judgment and should be determined on a case-by-case basis.

CHAPTER 5

Cultural Formulation

One of the improved elements of the DSM-5 is the updating of the Cultural Formulation Interview. In addition to acknowledging the impact culture has on behavior, this edition of the DSM calls for systematic assessment of the cultural identity of the individual, how that individual and his/her family conceptualizes distress, the key stressors experienced, the cultural features of vulnerability and resilience for the individual, how culture informs or interferes with the therapeutic relationship, and an overall cultural assessment (APA, 2013).

Development of the concept of culture as a contributor to mental illness is not new. Since the publication of the DSM-III in 1978, clinicians have been taught to explore how culture influences beliefs and behaviors. The DSM-5 expands the notion of "culture-bound syndromes" introduced in the DSM-III and explicitly defines terms and clarifies that: "Understanding the cultural context of illness experience is essential for effective diagnostic assessment and clinical management." (APA, 2013, p. 749).

DEFINITIONS OF TERMS

The DSM-5 draws a distinction between "race" and "ethnicity". The authors note that race has no consistent biological definition. Rather, it is based on a variety of "superficial physical traits" (APA, 2013, p. 749). These traits, when used to support ideological beliefs, racism, and discriminatory and social exclusion, have an adverse impact on the psychological and emotional well-being of individuals, families, and support systems.

Ethnicity is rooted in common histories, geography, language, customs and other shared group characteristics. These elements, separately or together, are used to distinguish one group from another. In determining group membership, individuals may be identified as belonging to a single group or having membership in a number of ethnic groups. The latter is typically due to inter-marriage and/or inter-mixing of cultures due to migration, immigration, or relocation due to war, environmental events, or economic pressures. All these combined also contribute to issues of identity, exclusion or inclusion, and other psychological issues of belonging (APA, 2013).

Culture is a meta concept that includes aspects of race and ethnicity, and, when looked at as a system, operates to preserve, transmit, and adapt knowledge, rules, values, and concepts across generations. These broad areas more specifically include language, religion and spiritual beliefs, practices and customs, family structure, identified developmental stages, moral and legal systems, and ceremonies and rituals that connect both individuals and groups. Cultures are typically thought of as being open, dynamic systems that respond to both internal and external forces. Individuals may belong to, participate in, and derive benefit from, multiple cultures. The DSM-5 explicitly cautions clinicians against overgeneralizing or stereotyping individuals and groups in terms of fixed cultural traits.

CULTURAL CONCEPTS OF DISTRESS

Psycho-physiologic distress may be experienced by all mammals, but expression of that distress entails great variability (Sopolsky, 1998; So, 2008; Tseng & Streltzer, 2008). Culture plays a pivotal role in how individuals, families, and family support networks experience, understand, communicate, and seek help around events and beliefs that they find distressing.

Expressions of distress within a culture consist of cultural and family norms. As such, these may be expressed on a continuum from "normal" to "abnormal", as these are understood within that culture. Where individuals or families find themselves outside of their culture, these expressions of distress may be misinterpreted or experienced differently, and thus labeled differently by observers and the individuals themselves. Systematically and respectfully exploring the cultural antecedents of distress is useful for building therapeutic rapport and positively influencing outcomes. Disregard of these variables may result in exacerbation of symptoms, disengagement from treatment, or psychopathologizing a culturally-appropriate response.

It is important to state explicitly that help-seeking behaviors typically arise only after many other strategies have been attempted and failed. As a provider, my sensitivity to and awareness of the cultural idioms of distress are threshold requirements for getting people the help they need.

CULTURAL FEATURES OF VULNERABILITY AND RESILIENCE

Adaptation to stressors appears to be part of our inherent design as mammals. Specific neurologic and physiologic responses mitigate the effects of external and internal stressors. When looked at solely through this individualistic lens, it is easy to discount or ignore the role of culture in contributing to vulnerability and resilience. This edition of the DSM opens that lens to specifically address the key stressors and supports in the individual and/or family's social environment. It acknowledges that this may include both proximal and distal events, and although not explicitly stated, these events should be explored both inter-generationally and across time.

Specifically looking at cultural interpretations of events, family structure, developmental tasks, and social context can provide clinicians with alternative explanations for behaviors and symptoms. Using strength-based approaches can positively impact the therapeutic relationship and outcomes of therapy. Accessing culturally-appropriate systems of support may result in healing more than just the individual symptoms.

Vulnerability to illness may be exacerbated by cultural dissonance, expectations, and chronic experiences of violence, poverty, racism, as well as environmental issues such as famine, exposure to chemicals, and climate-related catastrophes (Kirmayer, Dandeneau, Marshall, Phillips, & Williamson, 2011). Clinicians may not be aware of the exposure to these variables, and clients may not relate their experiences with them. A systematic evaluation of these possibilities may provide clues as to both risk and response to a variety of interventions, including culturally-derived customs and rituals that may not be within the traditional approach of the provider (Stumblingbear-Riddle, & Romans, 2012).

CULTURAL ISSUES BETWEEN PROVIDER AND CLIENT

Our work is based on establishing a trusting, respectful healing relationship that is focused on alleviating or diminishing the symptoms our clients are experiencing. The primary tools used are our own experience, training, and desire to help. Identifying differences not just in language, but also in social status, belief systems, and values must be done conscientiously and with care and respect. Failure to do so will most likely negatively impact therapeutic rapport, and may cause difficulties with diagnosis and treatment.

None of us is "culture-neutral". Our prejudices, values, beliefs, experiences with power, authority, class, and gender all influence our diagnostic approach. While we are expected to address these issues through training, continuing education, and self-exploration, unless we have access to other cultures and set an intention to address our own culturally-informed values and beliefs, we will be influenced by our own culture in our thinking and conclusions of someone else's behaviors and symptoms.

In spite of our best intentions, our clients' experiences with racism and discrimination in their own lives may adversely impact our capacity to connect with and provide treatment to them. Past experiences with institutions and individuals may influence expectations of treatment and care that interfere with addressing current problems. A sad illustration of this was the response to Hurricane Katrina in New Orleans in August of 2005.

The weather-driven crisis resulted in systems of care being overwhelmed, people being displaced geographically, and cultural support systems that were generations old not being able to be accessed. Well-intentioned volunteers found themselves unable to understand the Cajun culture and New Orleans Ward systems. The volunteers themselves were adversely affected by the experiences they had. Cultural misunderstandings resulted in individuals being denied psychological support as well as economic support. A long history of institutional racism and prejudice exacerbated the lack of facilities and support. Families were split up, neighborhoods were eviscerated, and reunification continues, some eight years later.

Without the CFI, information on these experiences might be overlooked or undervalued when seeing a client in another geographical setting. Many Katrina victims were bused to different communities across the country. Some stayed. In seeking assistance from their new communities, some individuals were assessed as having experienced depression and anxiety, but the additional burden of being displaced was not adequately evaluated. With the CFI, this can be systematically explored.

OVERALL CULTURAL ASSESSMENT

Once gathered, the information obtained from this exploration of culture can be used to inform treatment and management. This is not a pronouncement regarding the role that culture will play in the work, rather it is foundation from which the collaboration will emerge. Clinicians may need to address the client's experiences of prejudice BEFORE a treatment plan can be constructed. We may need to address beliefs about Western medicine and ego-based interventions that are in conflict with the client's cultural norms and values. We may benefit from including elders and healers, as well as rituals and ceremonies from the client's cultural support systems.

The next section goes through each component of the Cultural Formulation Interview in depth. It also discusses supplementary questions that can be used for follow-up.

Cultural Formulation Interview

The Cultural Formulation Interview (CFI) is a brief (16-question), semi-structured interview used to elicit the individual's experience, as well as inviting informants from that individual's social and cultural networks to contribute their observations. Four areas are explored using person-centered and problem-centered language. A script is provided to guide the interviewer in eliciting the client's cultural definition of the problem, his or her cultural perceptions as to the cause and context of the problem, as well as what support exists, what cultural factors affect the client's self-coping abilities and past help-seeking strategies, and what problems exist in terms of current help-seeking strategies.

Information may be sought from the client, or family members, or members of the client's extended community[2]. Supplementary modules are also available to use for gathering more in-depth information as well as for adjuncts to the 16-item CFI. Demographic information can be used to tailor the CFI questions to the client's specific background and current situation. DSM-5 authors suggest that the CFI is of particular assistance where there are significant cultural, religious, or socio-economic differences between therapist and client, or if there is uncertainty about diagnostic criteria and culturally distinctive symptoms. It may also be useful in determining severity and/or impairment. Where there is disagreement between the treatment provider and the client, the CFI may open up conversation. This might also be true in instances where there is perceived resistance to an intervention or treatment approach.

The interview provides guides for the interviewer as well as a specific script for each question. The script is well-written, and is useful as a training

---

[2] The reader may be wondering how information like this is gathered and/or shared, given HIPAA and confidentiality constraints. Many individuals who have experienced political targeting or persecution may have low tolerance for our regulatory requirements regarding obtaining releases of information. It is here that the clinician needs to use clinical judgment. At a minimum, attempts should be made to obtain releases of information. But it may be clinically contraindicated or therapeutically damaging to attempt to secure releases. Documenting why you did or did not get a release signed may be sufficient for the clinical record. It is prudent for clinicians to consult with risk management and other professional groups or seek supervision when working with these issues.

aid for students, interns, and even more experienced clinicians. The guide provides a linguistic and cultural context for asking the questions. There are no right or wrong answers for the CFI, and there is no scoring protocol.

Supplementary Modules

The 11 supplementary modules explore the CFI domains in depth. They can be accessed at: http://www.psychiatry.org/practice/dsm/dsm5/online-assessment-measures#Cultural. The first module looks at the client's way of explaining what is happening to him or her. Areas explored include the general understanding of the problem, what their illness prototype is, whether they have any causal explanation of what is happening, what they believe to be the course of their problem, and what they are hoping for from the help-seeking and treatment.

Cultural Issues

The second module looks at how cultural issues affect the client's level of functioning. It consists of eight questions that explore how the problem interferes with the client's ability to engage in daily activities of living, interact with family and others, and work, as well as overall financial situation, community participation, and enjoyment of everyday life. The final two questions ask the client to identify which of these issues is of most concern to him or her, and which is of most concern to others in their life.

Social Network

The third module explores the client's social network. There are 15 questions that look at who is in the client's social network and how that network interprets and/or explains the client's problem. It also looks at how the social network acts as a buffer and/or responds to the client's problem. Finally, it explores how the social network can be integrated into the treatment of the problem.

Client Stressors

The fourth module explores the client-identified stressors in depth. There are five questions that can be used to look at each stressor identified by the client. This module acknowledges that there may be culturally-related beliefs and constraints in sharing this very sensitive information. The first question asks about difficulties with family, work, money, or something else that may have made the problem worse. Subsequent questions ask about how others around the client cope with these issues, as well as how the client copes. The final two questions ask about what others have suggested in terms of addressing these issues, as well as what else could be done.

Spirituality, Religion, and Moral Traditions

The next module looks at spirituality, religious, and moral traditions and how these influence the client's problems and related stresses. There are 16 questions broken into four categories: 1) spiritual, moral, and religious identity, 2) the role of spiritual, religious, and moral values in the client's life, and that of his/her family and community, 3) relationship to the problem, and 4) potential stresses or conflicts related to spirituality, religion, and moral traditions.

Cultural Identity

The cultural identity module looks at how the problem may have been constructed. "Culture" is broadly defined here to include, "all the ways the individual understands his or her identity and experience in terms of groups, communities or other collectivities, including national or geographic origin, ethnic community, racialized categories, gender, sexual orientation, social class, religion/spirituality, and language" (APA 2013, CFI-Supplementary Interviews, p. 6). This is the longest of the modules, with 36 questions provided covering ethnic background, language, migration, spirituality, gender identity, and sexual orientation identity.

Coping and Help-Seeking

The next module explores how people may relate their problems in terms of symptoms, situations, and/or relationships. This module further investigates how the client has attempted to deal with these. Four areas are investigated: self-coping, using the social network, expanding beyond the social network (e.g., primary care doctor, mental health, spiritual/traditional healers), and more specifics about the current treatment episode (e.g., what brings you here today?).

Client-Provider Relationship

The eighth module focuses on the client/provider relationship, specifically on the experiences with and expectations of ways of communicating, and possible collaboration with the treatment provider. The word "patient" is used here in the module, most likely a vestige of the more hierarchical and traditional 'doctor-patient' relational model. Clinicians are invited to use appropriate language to more sensitively address the situation.

Children and Adolescents

Developmental issues are addressed in the school-age children and adolescents module. This consists of 20 questions, as well as a parental interview addendum. It is recommended that this be used in conjunction with standard child mental health assessments that evaluate family relations (including intergenerational issues), peer relations, and school environment. These questions identify the role of age-related cultural expectations, the possible cultural divergences between school, home, and the peer group, and whether these issues impact the situation or problem that brought the youth for care from the perspective of the child/youth. There are questions that indirectly explore cultural challenges, stressors and resilience, as well as issues of cultural hybridity, mixed ethnicity or multiple ethnic identifications. (APA, 2013, CFI-Supplemental, p. 10).

Instructions suggest that belonging is important to children and adolescents, and questions exploring peer group, ethnicity, religious identity, racism or gender difference should be asked following the child's lead. It further acknowledges that some children may not be able to answer all questions and encourages clinicians to select and adapt questions as developmentally appropriate. There is an explicit instruction that children not be used as informants for providing socio-demographic information on their family or an "explicit analysis of the cultural dimensions of their problems." (APA, 2013, CFI-Supplemental, p. 10).

Parental Addendum

The parental addendum lists cultural aspects of development and parenting that can be evaluated during interviews with parents, guardians, or caregivers. It consists of eight questions for follow-up, including birth-order, naming, developmental milestones, age-appropriate behaviors, relationships with adults, gender identity, languages spoken at home and outside the home, and spiritual aspects of home life.

CFI for Older Adults

There is also a module for older adults. These 17 questions look at how the client views his/her process of aging and at age-related transitions as they relate to this problem. Areas covered include conceptions of aging and cultural identity, conceptions of aging as related to illness attributions and coping, influence of comorbid medical problems and treatments on illness or problem, quality and nature of social supports and caregiving, additional age-related transitions, positive and negative attitudes towards aging, and the clinician-client relationship. This is more medically-focused, noting that for many older adults, coping with illness is the focus of their help-seeking.

Immigrants

The last of the modules can be used with individuals who are self-identified as immigrants and/or refugees. This module acknowledges that individuals and families may have experienced stressful events in their countries of origin, including prolonged and sometimes invasive and/or politically-charged interviews by officials, that may bring up resistance and challenges in your ability to gather information.

It also acknowledges the need for appropriate translation. It has been my experience that a literal translation rather than a cultural translation of the intent of the questions is insufficient, and may interfere with the development of a trusting, supportive relationship. As noted in the child module, relying on children to translate for families is not recommended. Efforts should be made to employ individuals who are both bi-lingual and bi-cultural, as well as being sufficiently trained to the nature and purpose of the interview.

Questions in this module explore the individual's background in their home country, their pre-immigration experience, any migration-related losses and challenges, their ongoing relationship with their country of origin, challenges with resettlement, how any of these may have impacted their problem, and what their future hopes and dreams are.

Using This Information with Clients

The very nature of these questions can either promote the development of an open and trusting relationship with the treatment provider, or can create an experience of being "poked-and-prodded" if the interview is not conducted with sensitivity and respect. It is natural to wonder why a perfect stranger would want to know about family, spiritual beliefs, and/or experiences coming to this country, when the problem is that my children are not being respectful, or I am experiencing anxiety.

Taking a page from narrative therapy (White & Epston, 1990), this type of "interviewing of the problem" can be both liberating and enlightening. These types of questions allow the problem to be externalized in a problem-centered, not person-centered way. For more information on narrative therapy, readers should go to the Dulwich Centre website (www.dulwichcentre.com.au).

Using This Information with Other Professionals

The DSM-5 is explicit in suggesting that as clinicians we need to attend to the cultural interpretations of illness that our clients bring with them. Reasons for this include avoiding misdiagnosis, obtaining useful information, improving clinical rapport and engagement, and improving clinical efficacy. It goes on to say: "Once the disorder is diagnosed, the cultural terms and explanations should be included in case formulations; they may help clarify symptoms and etiological attributions that could otherwise be confusing. Individuals whose symptoms do not meet DSM criteria for a specific mental disorder may still expect and require treatment (APA, 2013, p. 759).

One of the challenges of living in a highly mobile society is the repetitive nature of information gathering done to provide mental health services. I may start out in my home town, travel to another place for school, leave home and move to another location, and then change jobs resulting in more moves. If I find myself seeking help from government programs or institutions, I will fill out lots and lots of forms. I will be seen by many different people, each of whom will have their own take on my situation. Add to this mix the cultural stressors of language, vulnerability, and social and power narratives, and the sharing of accurate information becomes very important.

Use of the CFI and the supplemental interviews is a standardized way to capture and share information that may actually be quite painful or stressful for our clients to reveal. Reducing the number of times that information is gathered may be therapeutic in and of itself.

Scoring and Interpretation

This is an interview, not a quantitative assessment. Thus, no answers are weighted or scores are obtained. Integrating what you have learned about your clients' cultural background and how that background influences, contributes to and/or protects against mental illness is where the art of diagnosis is applied.

Using the CFI may help avoid misdiagnosing behaviors or overly estimating severity of symptoms. For example, there are cultural expressions of grief that may look pathological or severe whereas they are appropriate when understood within the framework of the individual's culture. Another application is to clarify meanings, which if used idiomatically may construct an entirely different meaning than when used clinically. For example, the word "depression" carries different connotations when describing a clinical syndrome, discussing things with friends on social media, or identifying a source of behavior.

Perhaps the fundamental benefit of using the CFI is to establish clinical rapport and engagement. Using the client's words, metaphors, and concepts will improve communication, satisfaction, information-sharing, and hopefully sustain the changes that the client is looking for from therapy and your work together.

CONCLUSION

Incorporating a cultural evaluation of a client's functioning into treatment planning and diagnosis is essential to achieving positive outcomes. Cultural information can be gathered systematically and with sensitivity using the CFI and the supplemental modules. Whether done by a clinician or other staff member, the information gathered can go a long way in establishing trust and good therapeutic rapport.

Sharing of the information with other treatment providers can assist to ensure that clients in our highly mobile society are not unduly burdened with having to undergo potential re-traumatization in telling their story. The information may also provide a better understanding of behavior, adaptation strategies, and levels of support needed to restore optimal functioning.

Finally, the CFI is an excellent model of taking a good clinical history as well as providing opportunities to use culturally-specific language to externalize the problem and join with the client in a respectful and therapeutically sensitive way. This will benefit students, interns, and more seasoned clinicians alike.

CHAPTER 6

Alternative Model for Personality Disorders

The DSM-5 has fundamentally changed how we look at the constellation of symptoms and behaviors that constitute human 'being-ness'. One of the more challenging areas to pin down are personality disorders. The DSM-5 work group for this area struggled mightily with accommodating the shift from symptom-specific diagnosis to dimensional diagnosis, ultimately unable to reach a compromise and instead settling on offering clinicians two models. The DSM-IV model of 12 symptom-specific diagnoses remains in the DSM-5 without any changes. A hybrid, alternative model based on evaluation of traits and functioning, however, is found in Section III.

This alternative model offers much, and I am hopeful that it will replace what has been standard for over 30 years. The following looks at how aspects of the alternative model can be used in working with individuals who experience disruption and/or distress in functioning due to trait pathology.

HISTORY AND DEVELOPMENT

What appears to be a radical change in evaluation and determination of personality disorders is actually less so when looked at systematically. Members of the Personality Disorders Work group proposed these changes as far back as 2004 at a conference held in Arlington, Virginia. The "Future of Psychiatric Diagnosis: Refining the Research Agenda" series included 23 invited participants representing the United States and other nations who presented papers focused on the diagnosis and classification of Personality Disorders.

Presenters looked at limitations of the categorical model, biologic and genetic ways of looking at personality dimensions, the neuroscience of emotionality, personality dimensions across cultures, the underlying structure of personality and how it manifests in terms of traits and behaviors, coverage (i.e., whether the system adequately characterizes conditions that are encountered in clinical practice) and cutoffs (i.e., how to make the judgment that personality pathology is sufficiently severe to warrant clinical attention), and finally, clinical utility.

Dimensional Models of Personality

Dimensional models of personality functioning and disorders have been studied for years. A dimensional model for personality disorders was considered for inclusion in the DSM-IV, but was ultimately rejected because of competing and incompatible models, lack of empirical data regarding validity, and questions about the clinical utility of a dimensional system.

According to the personality disorders work group (First, 2004):

> The goal of this conference, therefore, was to stimulate research toward the development of a dimensional model of personality disorder that would have a strong empirical foundation with respect to behavioral genetics, neurobiological mechanisms, childhood antecedents, cross-cultural application, continuity with the rest of the diagnostic manual, coverage of clinical relevant maladaptive personality functioning, diagnostic thresholds, and treatment implications.

Although much research was evaluated and many meetings held, the work group was not successful in lobbying the APA community to replace the current categorical evaluation of these disorders. Instead, an unholy compromise of setting both out in the same book was arrived at.

CLINICAL ISSUES AND PRACTICAL CONSIDERATIONS

The alternative model for diagnosing personality disorders is clinically very useful. It is a three-step process that results in identification of functioning on a continuum, and anticipates the variability of traits and expressions of pathology, rather than categorically labeling the individual.

Coding

The practical aspects of implementing the model rest in deciding how to code for the disorder(s). Essentially, coding will not change, and all 12 of the personality disorders contained in the DSM-IV remain. Thus, if you have a client who has an included DSM-IV personality disorder (e.g., paranoid, histrionic, or dependent), you would continue to code for that on your insurance claims, but you would have the option of evaluating the individual's functioning using the DSM-5 evaluation methodology. Roel Verheul, PhD., a presenter at the 2004 conference, argued that:

> . . .a dimensional diagnostic system will substantially improve clinical utility, especially with respect to coverage, reliability, subtlety (i.e., level of detail and richness) and clinical decision making. . . . however, whatever dimensional model is chosen in the future, it cannot entirely replace a categorical system, which will continue to be needed for legal, medical, and administrative purposes (p. 283).

His comments presaged the final publication of the DSM-5.

LEVELS OF PERSONALITY FUNCTIONING

The DSM-5 alternative model suggests that two determinations must be met when diagnosing a personality disorder: level of impairment and evaluation of which personality traits are pathological in nature. Disturbances in "self" and "interpersonal functioning" are hallmarks of personality disorders. The alternative model suggests that these disturbances are best evaluated on a continuum, rather than on a dichotomous, "present/not present" scale.

"Self" is further divided into elements of identity and self-direction. The DSM-5 provides definitions of both these. "Identity" consists of the individual's experience of self and other, including self-esteem and capacity for and ability to regulate emotions. "Self-direction" includes the ability to have and pursue life goals, to have internalized standards of behavior that are constructive and pro-social, and to be able to be self-reflective.

Interpersonal functioning is also bifurcated specifically identifying empathy and intimacy as measurable elements. "Empathy" is defined as having both comprehension and appreciation of the experiences and motivations of others, as well as understanding the effects of behavior on others. "Intimacy" consists of connection, closeness, and regard, as evidenced by depth and duration of the connection, desire and capacity for closeness, and mutuality reflected in interpersonal behavior.

Diagnostic Process

To diagnose a personality disorder, clinicians must first evaluate these domains and then identify whether there is an impairment and then finally determine the severity of that impairment. The DSM-5 suggests the threshold level for a personality disorder is a moderate level of impairment. Table 2 on pages 775 through 778 in the DSM-5 provides descriptors for the levels of functioning ranging from "0" (little or no impairment) to "4" (extreme impairment). Descriptions are provided across the domains (self and interpersonal) and within the subdomains of identity and self-direction and empathy and intimacy. These are well-written and very understandable and can be used for treatment planning or disability determination.

These initial evaluations determine levels of personality functioning. This alone, however, does not complete the diagnosis. Clinicians must also identify which of the personality traits are pathologic, the pervasiveness of the traits and stability of functioning, and then rule out alternative explanations.

LEVELS OF PATHOLOGY

Drawing from the Five-Factor Model (FFM) of personality, the DSM-5 alternative model identifies the following pathological personality traits: detachment, antagonism, disinhibition, and psychoticism. Within these domains they identify 25 specific trait facets shown in the table below. Definitions for these traits and facts can be found in the DSM-5 on pages 779-781.

Table 7   Alternative Model for Personality Disorders: Trait Domains and Facets

Negative Affectivity	Detachment	Antagonism	Disinhibition	Psychoticism
Emotional Lability	Withdrawal	Manipulativeness	Irresponsibility	Unusual beliefs and experiences
Anxiousness	Intimacy avoidance	Deceitfulness	Impulsivity	Eccentricity
Separation insecurity	Anhedonia	Grandiosity	Distractibility	Cognitive and perceptual dysregulation
Submissiveness	Depressivity	Attention-seeking	Risk-taking	
Hostility	Restricted affectivity	Callousness	Rigid perfectionism (lack of)	
Perseveration	Suspiciousness	Hostility		
Depressivity				
Suspiciousness				
Restricted affectivity (lack of)				

Diagnostic Criteria

Diagnostic criteria for the specific personality disorders consists of seven items: 1) moderate or greater impairment in personality functioning, 2) identification of the specific personality traits that are pathologic, 3) demonstration that the impairments are relatively inflexible and pervasive across a broad range of personal and social situations, 4) these impairments and trait expression are "relatively stable" and have an onset at least at adolescence or early adulthood, 5) these impairments and traits can't be explained by something else (e.g., culture, circumstance, illness), 6) these can't be attributed to the physiological effects of a substance or medical condition (e.g., head trauma), and 7) these are not better understood as "normal" for the developmental stage or sociocultural environment. (APA, 2013, p. 761).

Personality Disorder-Trait-Specific

Each of the six personality disorders proposed in the alternative model consists of "typical features", specific descriptions of impairment in identity, self-direction, empathy, and intimacy, and descriptions of disorder-specific pathological personality traits. An additional diagnosis of Personality Disorder—Trait Specified (PD-TS) is proposed for individuals where a personality disorder is considered present, but the criteria are not fully met. For this diagnosis, the clinician would note the severity of impairment in personality functioning and the problematic personality trait(s).

PRACTICAL APPLICATIONS

Since the alternative model was *not* adopted, clinicians should continue to use the categorical criteria found on pages 645 through 684 of the DSM-5 for coding purposes. With that said, I would encourage clinicians and supervisors to incorporate aspects of the dimensional evaluation into treatment planning and training of clinicians. There is great value in systematically looking at how an individual manages the complexities of self-identity and interpersonal connections. Exploring which areas are problematic, rather than labeling an individual as "Axis II" or "personality-disordered" is far more beneficial.

THE CHALLENGE OF DIAGNOSING PERSONALITY DISORDERS

In my classroom work and in supervision, I have noticed that diagnosing personality disorders can be quite challenging. Many of my students suggest that they can qualitatively identify aspects of functioning that are problematic for the individual. While this may indicate high levels of intuition and sensitivity, it does not support the requirements for validity and reliability to which the DSM ascribes. This intuitive metric is not limited to behavioral health practitioners. According to a study done by Commons and Lewis (2009), there is a tendency across professions to become distracted by certain behaviors, (for example cutting in borderline personality disorder), and then derive the diagnosis from that alone. This is not *good* clinical practice, but it is, unfortunately, common clinical practice.

Categorical vs. Dimensional

When using categorical criteria alone rather than dimensional evaluations, clinicians and students may find themselves in the morass of determining whether a specific trait (i.e., suspiciousness) is attributable to a pattern of interpersonal interaction (avoidant personality disorder) or another pattern of behavior (e.g., prolonged marijuana use). In addressing these kinds of differential diagnostic challenges, the DSM-5 notes, "It may be particularly difficult (and not particularly useful) to distinguish personality disorders from persistent mental disorders such as persistent depressive disorder that have an early onset and an enduring, relatively stable course." (APA, 2013, p. 648).

These examples are for illustrative purposes only. Readers can reflect on their own experience, understanding, and preferred methods of arriving at a diagnosis. My point is that quantifying behaviors that are intrinsically qualitative in nature is challenging at best. Systematic evaluation of functioning in specific domains goes a long way toward supporting a more objective conclusion and diagnosis.

Criticisms of Dimensional Model

One of the criticisms of the alternative model and its predecessor is that it is too cumbersome. I have experienced the challenges of trying to explain the methodology to seasoned clinicians as well as to students. Where the problem appears to lie is in determining what is problematic for the individual client. By definition, a personality disorder is an "enduring pattern of inner experience and behavior . . ." (APA, 2013, p. 646). The individual may not experience this pattern or inner experience as being problematic, even though the balance of the definition requires that it ". . .deviates markedly from the expectations of the individual's culture" (APA, 2013, p. 646).

Thus, the clinician must first determine whether there is any impairment. This is a moderately objective task that requires interviewing the client, obtaining information from collaterals, and then exploring with the client how they believe the impairment causes problems. After that is done, the clinician must then determine which traits identified are problematic. Once that is done, a final evaluation of the degree of impairment can be made.

For those of us trained in the categorical method, our work used be done after the first pass. In the alternative model, we are asked to re-visit the information and take the additional step of exploring functioning in finer detail. This is not unusual in research settings, but it may be a luxury for clinicians who are working with emergent situations or who do not have the opportunity to develop long-term relationships with a client.

Measuring Functional Variability

Once the methodology becomes familiar, however, the evaluation becomes less cumbersome and results in more than just a diagnosis. It results in clearly defined areas that are measurable in terms of monitoring for change and determining the success of outcomes. This is a benefit to both client and practitioner. Further, the alternative model allows for more frequent evaluation of functioning than the categorical approach, assuming, as it does, that the individual will experience some variation in functioning even though a trait or several traits may be present and problematic at any given time.

The alternative model potentially allows for greater cohesiveness in cross-provider treatment and interventions. For example, a client diagnosed with borderline personality disorder may be seen by a psychiatrist for medications, a psychologist for assessment, a social worker for resources, a case manager for day-to-day issues, emergency room staff when impulsive, a psychiatric nurse for aftercare, a group treatment team for partial-day hospitalization and intensive out-patient treatment, substance treatment specialists and a primary care physician for non-psychiatric issues. It is possible for each of these treatment providers to see a different level of functional impairment, yet each will provide essentially the same diagnosis. Clinical utility surely lies more in the realm of the distinctions in functioning than in solely meeting the criteria for the categorical diagnosis.

USING THE INFORMATION WITH CLIENTS

Because there is such stigma attached to having a personality disorder, we need to carefully approach sharing our insights and conclusions. What may be useful to us, may be experienced by a client as labeling or worse. Alternatively, it may be enlightening for a client to think about how they are interacting with the world in terms of traits, self-direction, intimacy, and empathy. The alternative model provides language that describes levels of functioning in terms of the four domains and in terms of severity. This dimensional approach is more descriptive of the variability of functioning within individuals. For example, using the Level of Personality Functioning Scale (LPFS), a client may be experiencing little or no impairment in the domain of identity, but have moderate impairment in terms of self-direction. Simultaneously, depending on situational factors, that same client may experience severe impairment in empathy, and some impairment in intimacy.

Specific descriptors for each of these levels is found in the LPFS. These can be explored with the client to see if they are accurately describing the client's current experience. Plotting changes over time may be useful for determining patterns and/or contributing factors to changes in functioning. The chart below shows functioning of a client of mine with borderline personality disorder over a period of six months. My client was a high-functioning 45 year-old professional. She initially came to see me about her anxiety and lack of focus in her life. After a few sessions, it became evident to me that there were personality traits that were interfering with her functioning. I approached the notion of her having a personality disorder and she reacted strongly. For her, the label was both hurtful and damaging. When I reframed it as a functional impairment, she was more open to seeing how these aspects of her self-concept contributed to her overall feelings of being different. Once she accepted the

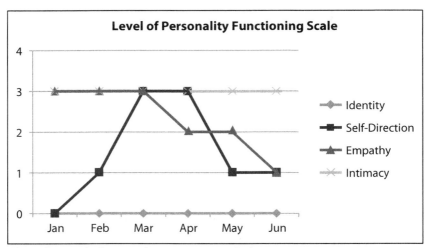

Chart 6   Level of Personality Functioning Scale

Note: Functional impairment of 2 or higher on the y axis is required.

reframe, she made good use of the distinctions between self and inter-personal functioning. This led to a better understanding of the variability of functioning in her life and allowed us to collaborate on interventions and strategies to better address her needs.

Functional Impairment Threshold

Clinicians should note that the diagnosis of a personality disorder in the DSM-5 alternative model requires a functional impairment of moderate or greater in at least two of the domains. It may also be used as a more global indicator of personality functioning, especially where there is insufficient evidence for a full diagnosis.

We would check in once a month using the scale to identify how my client had been doing. The scale focused our conversation to these areas, which my client reported as being beneficial primarily because she often felt overwhelmed and unable to speak specifically about her experience. Focusing on her functioning rather than her symptoms helped her to put her experience on a continuum where she could see the variability in some areas and the stability in others.

PERSONALITY INVENTORIES

If you go to the DSM-5 website, you can download personality inventories (both short and long forms) for adults and children ages 11 to 17. These can be used to identify pathological traits and domain functioning. Each instrument is described below in detail.

As noted in Chapter 4, training in administering, scoring, and interpreting tests and measures is NOT typically part of medical education, and only a small part of training in most master's level programs. At first glance, it may appear that it is easy to administer and score the personality inventories, but I would challenge that assumption and encourage all clinicians to follow the applicable ethical guidelines regarding limitations in administering or interpreting tests and measures they may be subject to.

Cautions Regarding Use of Personality Assessments in DSM-5

The area of personality assessment is a domain that has been limited to psychologists and psychological assessment for many decades. The DSM-5 appears to be entering into that domain without adequately addressing the interpretation of the results of these personality measures. This is both an ethical and professional dilemma. The inventory found on the website is quite similar to the Minnesota Multiphasic Personality Inventory (MMPI), considered the gold standard in personality assessment. Psychology graduate students typically take at least one if not several courses on the administration, scoring and interpretation of this instrument. There is no such expectation, or supporting documentation, for the DSM-5 version. This is a substantial clinical weakness and suggests that you take time to consider whether this is a useful instrument to use. At a minimum, before you entertain the notion of using these measures, I would review any training you have had in tests and measures, particularly as it relates to the evaluation of personality. I would include caveats in the reporting of results, particularly if you are not a psychologist trained in the administration and interpretation of results.

The Personality Inventory for DSM-5 (PID-5)—Adult

This inventory consists of 220 questions and provides scores for 25 personality trait facets grouped into five personality trait domains. While it mirrors similar information found in the Minnesota Multiphasic Personality Inventory (the granddaddy of all personality inventories), it differs in that it uses the "Big Five" personality traits as indicators and assesses using a 4-point Likert scale rather than 'True/False'. Results are shown in terms of raw facet scores, total facet scores, and total facet domain scores.

The challenge of this inventory is its length. Respondents may not have the attentional capacity or willingness to complete all the questions. In that case, a shorter version is available and is discussed below. There is an informant version provided which may also be used.

Scoring

As one can imagine, the scoring for this instrument is complex. Instructions are provided but may be confusing for some. Readers can download Excel spreadsheets from *go.pesi.com/DSM-5* at no cost. This requires inputting some results by hand. There may be other ways of doing this or someone may be designing an app even as you read this! A domain chart is provided below to illustrate information that you can use with your client. This client's responses would suggest that there is not a personality disorder, but there are two trait domains (disinhibition and negative affect) that warrant further exploration because their scores are approaching the threshold of "2" or mild).

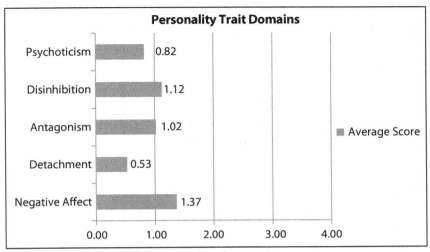

Chart 7 Personality Trait Domains Results

The Personality Inventory for DSM-5—Informant Form (PID-5-IRF)—Adult is essentially the same as the adult form, but is answered by a "knowledgeable other". This would appropriately be a caregiver, family member, or friend who knows the client well. This form would be useful for times where the client is unable and/or unwilling to complete the inventory as well as for obtaining collateral information.

Interpretation

Sophisticated evaluation of the results, similar to what can be obtained through administration of the MMPI, is not available using this instrument. Thus, caution should be used when drawing conclusions. Additionally, until further data are gathered as to the accuracy and content validity of the facets and domains, it is unlikely that these instruments would be considered for forensic use.

The Personality Inventory for DSM-5—Brief Form (PID-5-BF)—Adult

This version takes the longer, full version and selects five representative questions for each of the five trait domains. As with the full version, clinicians can gauge functioning on a 4-point Likert scale. This is a more manageable inventory because of its short length, however, it does not provide the same level of detail.

Scoring

Answers are summed for an overall score (0-75), with higher scores indicating greater problems with functioning. Individual domain scores can also be calculated by averaging the answers to the five questions within each domain. Excel spreadsheets can be found at *go.pesi.com/DSM-5* with formulas for calculating these scores provided. If more than two questions are left unanswered in any domain, that domain score should not be calculated. If more than seven questions are left blank, the inventory should not be scored.

Personality Inventory for Children and Adolescents Ages 11-17 – Long and Brief Forms

These are exactly the same as the PID for Adults. While there are psychometric shortcomings in doing this, it makes administration and scoring straightforward. Caution should be used, however, in interpreting results, as the DSM website does not provide information on norms or standard deviations for this population. As with the PID-Adult form, a spreadsheet with scoring is provided in the forms section.

CONCLUSION

It is not clear when, if ever, the alternative model for personality functioning will be adopted. There is great benefit, however, in reading through and exploring this way of assessing functioning and distress for individuals who have personality disorders. The personality inventories provided on the DSM-5 website may be useful in helping clinicians and clients alike to identify and explore specific trait facets that interfere with inter- and intra-personal functioning. Administering and scoring the inventories can be a bit confusing and even burdensome. While these may not be used as frequently as other measures, they can provide evidence as well as verbiage to address issues raised in determining disability.

Clinicians should continue to use the coding of personality disorders found in the chapter on personality disorders. The alternative model has not yet been officially adopted. Alternative assessments that have been standardized and well-researched are still preferred.

CHAPTER 7

Group Practice and Agency Issues

Having worked in a non-profit agency, I have come to appreciate that implementing change is challenging. There are so many variables! With the changes to the DSM-5, there is an excellent opportunity to enhance quality aspects of service provision. These measures are tailored to several quality improvement goals—the performance improvement project (PIP), outcomes analysis, and monitoring change.

I realize these elements are frequently resisted and or resented by hardworking clinicians in the public and private sector. That aside, taking a look at how and what you are doing and asking if it can be done in a better, more effective way, is an essential business strategy. With the advent of the Affordable Care Act, all providers will need to consistently evaluate their performance.

An unanticipated benefit of the Level-2 Cross-Cutting Symptom measures is that these are ready-made for performance improvement projects and monitoring effectiveness of change. They are brief, use an accepted quantifiable scale, are free, and have good test-retest reliability. What is necessary is understanding how the measures need to be utilized, how staff need to be oriented and trained in their use, and policy and procedures written to accommodate use.

It is not the purpose of this book to educate you on how to design a quality improvement project. Rather, this chapter will outline the steps necessary to incorporate these (and other) measures into your agency.

THINGS TO CONSIDER

Getting buy-in from all stakeholders: While this seems obvious, because it is time-consuming and sometimes challenging, this step may be minimized or overlooked altogether. Stakeholders include consumers, clinicians, policymakers, fiscal and administrative personnel, and board members. Information may need to be provided in different formats to insure that all stakeholders understand what is being proposed. This takes time and assignment of sufficient resources to insure buy-in.

Providing training on what the measures measure: The information gathered is only as good as understanding what it means. Flour, eggs, butter, sugar and milk mean nothing without a recipe and measures of ingredients. With the recipe, you get a cake! Training people on each of the measures will go a long way towards ensuring the results justify all the time and effort needed.

Time-frame to monitor: Some of the measures can be used once. All can be used to measure more frequently. Deciding what you want to measure will usually indicate the frequency with which you need to administer one or more of the assessments. The more stable a trait, the less frequently it needs to be measured. Alternatively, if you are looking at program outcomes, you may wish to sample on a regular basis (e.g., monthly, quarterly, annually). A word of caution here, in some cases, discrete information may be lost within a longer period of evaluation (i.e., annually). More frequent sampling may result in odd spikes of results that, if looked at over a longer period of time, would even out. Determining the frequency of measuring is part of the CQI process. Using the measures in a pilot will go a long way in providing clues as to how frequently they can be used to gather the information that is desired.

How to gather and analyze results: In an agency or group setting, it is always advisable to use a pilot before committing fully to implementation of an evaluation program. This will help work out the kinks ahead of time. I have found it useful to establish a small group of collaborators that includes folks who love data, folks who detest it, and folks who are going to use it. This group can hash out the nuts and bolts of what works best in the specific work environment.

Many agencies have integrated using electronic media and hardware. While this is a large financial investment, it pays off in both accuracy of data gathered and security of the information. On the analysis end, downloading data from these machines is ever so much easier than hand entering into a computer. If the electronic route is not available due to fiscal reasons or technology constraints, data can still be gathered on paper and then entered into a data base.

One important consideration to make at the beginning is what kind of reports will be useful to the different stakeholders. This planning up front will make the data gathering more streamlined and its utility more accessible.

How to share results: Decisions need to be made at a policy level regarding what kinds of information will be shared and with whom. HIPAA regulations and state regulations guide this discussion and planning. Additional decisions need to be made in terms of what format results will be shared in and how long the information will be retained. Stakeholders play an important role in exploring this, and it is vital that their input be sought.

THE PILOT

In gathering information for this book, I called upon colleagues who work in local agencies and asked them to pilot the WHODAS. These agencies provide services to marginalized individuals who typically cannot afford private therapy. They meet the needs of children, families, and seriously and persistently mentally ill individuals in a moderately sized city in Northern California. Clients are typically economically marginalized, and frequently encounter levels of prejudice.

OBTAINING RESULTS

In order for the agencies to provide services, funding sources frequently require evidence that the monies provided are obtaining results. Using the WHODAS is one way to accomplish two goals: evaluating the impact of services on the targeted populations and obtaining this information using culturally and linguistically appropriate measures.

Systematically gathering WHODAS information can provide agencies with data to illustrate the impact of their services individually and community-wide. Data are easily aggregated and can be used overtime to demonstrate adherence to mission and accomplishment of goals. It can also be an effective tool for fundraising.

IMPACT OF SERVICES

Many non-profits must demonstrate how their services change the lives of those they serve. Remembering that the WHODAS 2.0 looks at functioning in six domains, it should be clear to the reader that this instrument can provide evidence of change. The benefit here is that this information can be gathered as part of the clinical intake as well as during treatment and may augment the satisfaction surveys which are typically provided to consumers.[3]

---

[3] I must admit to a bias here. Having been involved in local, County, and state-level evaluations of services, I have come to the conclusion that satisfaction surveys are of little value. While they provide the dissatisfied consumer the opportunity of complaining, they typically provide results that show that 70% of the people are 'satisfied'. This does not help to improve a program, nor does it allow for a means to address the 30% for whom dissatisfaction was the experience.

In running this pilot, the program director identified questions to determine utility for clinicians. These questions were: Do you find the information obtained useful? Would you actually find it helpful in monitoring your clients? What things might be problematic in using it with your clients? What might you find supportive in using it with your clients? How would you rate the instrument's ease of use? How applicable is this instrument for working with the population you serve?

The pilot was implemented over a period of several weeks. Results were, on the whole, quite positive. From an administrative perspective, several steps needed to be taken before the measure was used. These included presenting to the agency's executive director, getting buy-in from the clinical director and staff, considering the implications in terms of privacy, research subject protection, and data security, and finally introducing the measure to the staff, deciding how and when it would be used and how the information would be collected.

Each of these steps is quite involved in and of itself. If this were to be done agency-wide and not just as a pilot, policies and procedures would have to be written and reviewed, trainings would need to be set up, and changes to computer systems, charting, etc., would need to be considered and addressed. All this costs time and money.

The question is: "Do the results support the investment of the time and money?" The answer will depend on how the agency views the information. If this is just another task that staff need to do, then there is little likelihood that the implementation of the change will be successful. On the other hand, if end-users (clients), staff, and supervisors see benefit and have a sense of ownership of the measures, then there is a greater likelihood for success.

USING THE INFORMATION

Using the information to make changes to how the work is done is just as important as gathering the information. There are several ways information from these measures can be used: justification for grant proposals; year-end reporting on performance; program description (both qualitative and quantitative).

PERFORMANCE IMPROVEMENT PROJECTS

The Level-2 symptom measures are custom-made for monitoring specific areas of practice. For example, using the adult-depression measure, you can identify all clients who carry a diagnosis of major depressive disorder, single episode, mild (296.21/F32.0), identify a target sample, and measure change in functioning using several different interventions (e.g., changing appointment times, changing modality, changing medications).

The federal government has required states to identify performance improvements for over 30 years. State agencies and non-profits receiving funding through the state have been tasked with putting together these projects. In the agencies I have worked for, these typically are experienced as an added burden. Benefits of such projects frequently do not 'trickle-down' to front-line staff or clients.

There is the possibility with the implementation of both the WHO-DAS 2.0 and some (or all!) of the Level 1 and Level-2 symptom monitors, this information may prove useful to all stakeholders. For the first time, these standardized measures can be used to collect information at the client level, the agency level, the county level, and the state level, because of their standardization. From a program perspective, data may be valuable for obtaining funding, demonstrating improvement, and making the case for expanded services to individuals with mental illness. From a policy perspective, data may prove invaluable for demonstrating to non-mental health professionals that addressing the functioning of clients improves the welfare of all citizens, and is worthy of additional funding and support.

This is contingent on the planned implementation of use in an agency and governmental setting. Without buy-in from stakeholders and providers, this information will just be one more barrier to good clinical treatment. Because these measures are in the public domain, there are fewer barriers to implementation. Collecting and sharing the results does require modification of electronic health record coding and other considerations in terms of consistency of reporting of the data and collection and retention of the information. These are beyond the scope of this book.

CONCLUSION

All indicators suggest that delivery of behavioral health services is going toward a pay-for-performance model. NGOs and local government have long been tasked with providing evidence that what they do makes a difference in the lives of those they serve. Historically this has been done using self-report and satisfaction data. The DSM-5 contains instruments that I believe will enhance the gathering of information that not only show that our programs and interventions are changing lives for the better, but can help clinicians tailor services to meet the needs of those they serve. This is truly a Win-Win!

CHAPTER 8

Documentation and Billing Implications

If you use any of the measures discussed in this book, there is a good chance that you will need to document your time. What is not clear is whether you will be reimbursed for your efforts.

As a caveat, determinations for reimbursement are made based on the payer (e.g., Medicare, Blue Cross/Blue Shield, etc.). There are several procedural codes identified in the Current Procedural Terminology (CPT®) book published by the American Medical Association that suggest there may be possible reimbursement, but these are subject to interpretation and scope of practice issues. These are discussed in more detail below.

WHAT SHOULD YOU DOCUMENT?

There has been a standard of practice for decades that says raw data should not be shared with clients. With the recent changes in HIPAA, this standard is being challenged. Raw data, in and of itself, is typically not very useful to the uninitiated. An example of this is blood work. If you don't understand what the numbers mean, they are just numbers. You need context to understand what is considered to be "normal", "below normal" or "above normal." Similarly, when looking at behaviors on self-report measures, the numbers are only representative of what the individual interprets them to mean on the day s/he fills the measure out.

Far more useful is interpreting the results, and sharing that interpretation with your client. Keep in mind, interpretations are not "fact" or "truth". They are suggestive of meaning that needs to be confirmed with your client. This applies to information you share with your client in the patient/therapist relationship. Documentation of this may be subject to review by others, and you need to have an awareness of this when you include this information in the client's chart.

Here is a way to think through this: You have your work with your client. That consists of obtaining a:

> clinical history and concise summary of the social, psychological, and biological factors that may have contributed to developing a given mental disorder . . . using all available contextual and diagnostic information to develop a comprehensive treatment plan informed by the individual's cultural and social context. (APA 2013, p 19).

All that information needs to be documented in the client chart. This is just one element of documentation. Information obtained as the therapeutic relationship grows also goes in the chart. This includes the measures discussed in this book. Consistent documentation provides evidence of effective change and adherence to standards of practice. Should you ever need to substantiate your work, having a well-documented chart will go a long way in seeing you get paid.

Documenting Results

There is an axiom in auditing circles, "If you didn't write it down, it didn't happen." But how do you "write down" results from a measure such as the WHODAS or Level-1 and what do you say about it? Answers to some commonly asked questions and suggestions for charting follow.

Is the information being used to diagnose, treat, or communicate information to another treatment provider? If yes, then connect the measure to that specific thing. For example, if the Level-1 is being used to identify goals in a treatment plan, you would incorporate the results by saying, "reduce levels of anxiety and depression as evidenced in the Level-1 Cross Cutting Symptom Measure from severe to mild." In communicating information with another treatment provider, you might say, "client reports moderate and severe levels of impairment in 4 of 12 domains on the Level-1 Symptom Measure". If you are using it to diagnose, you might state: "Endorsement of severe levels of depression, anxiety, and personality functioning are consistent with individuals who have borderline personality disorder, as well as individuals who have bipolar disorder. Additional testing is indicated to determine an accurate diagnosis." There may be specific requirements in the worksite that would further limit or require additional information to be shared. In such cases, you will need to obtain a release of information or chart the reason why you did NOT obtain a release of information.

You might also document that you administered, scored or interpreted the measure and give a brief summary of the result. For example. "Saw client today. Reviewed results of Level-1 Symptom measure, noting client endorsed severe levels in depression and anxiety. Client states that he still is experiencing difficulty in these areas." An alternative entry might read, "Scored Level-1 Sx measure and provided written interpretation to client and primary care physician." If someone other than yourself is providing the information to the client, for example an intake coordinator, you would chart, "Client completed following measures at intake. Results reviewed with client."

Should you obtain authorization for using these from the payer in order to get paid? It is not clear whether these measures will be considered "psychological testing" as defined in the CPT® promulgated by the American Medical Association. This may be decided in the future.

Where should results be kept in a chart? This would be an important discussion to have with your records department if you are in an agency or group BEFORE you implement use of the measures.

What information should be included in the results? At a minimum, results should include the client name, date of administration, your name, and the record/account number. Additional information would include the specific name of the measure and, of course, your interpretation. You might also include a statement that cautions others about using the results. For example, "Information contained in this report is protected and confidential. Sharing or use by individuals other than the client or persons not authorized to participate in the treatment of the client is prohibited by federal regulations."

CONCLUSION

It is important to take time before you implement these measures to consider how you will share the information with your clients, where that information will be kept, and how you will be paid for what you do. These are variables that are outside the scope of this book. Practitioners will need to stay up to date with the changes coming due to the implementation of the Affordable Care Act (ACA), the Mental Health Parity Act (MHPA), documentation standards set by the Centers for Medicare and Medicaid, as well as insurance companies.

As these standards evolve, how you document will evolve. Consideration for keeping information in an electronic format is not addressed in the DSM-5. These, and other advances in technology, will affect how you record and share information.

References

Aggarwal, N. K., Nicasio, A. V., DeSilva, R., Boiler, M., & Lewis-Fernández, R., (2013). Barriers to implementing the DSM-5 cultural formulation interview: A qualitative study. *Culture, Medicine, and Psychiatry, 37*(3), 505-533.

American Psychiatric Association,(2000) *Diagnostic and statistical manual of mental disorders.* (4th ed., text revision). Washington, DC: Author

American Psychiatric Association (2013). *Diagnostic and statistical manual of mental disorders.* (5th ed). Washington, DC: Author.

Anonymous (2009). The patient reported outcomes measurement information system (PROMIS): A walk through the first four years. NIH: Washington, DC *www.nihpromis.org/measures/measureshome*

Baldwin, L., Keppel, G. A., Davis, A., Guirguis-Blake, J., Force, R. W., & Berg, A. O. (2012). Developing a practice-based research network by integrating quality improvement: Challenges and ingredients for success. *CTS: Clinical & Translational Science, 5*(4), 351-355.

Berman, P. S. (2009). Case conceptualization and treatment planning: Exercises for integrating theory with clinical practice. Thousand Oaks, CA. Sage Publications:

Brütt, A., Schulz, H., & Andreas, S. (2013). Development of an ICF-based core set of activities and participation for patients with mental disorders: an approach based upon data. *Clinical Rehabilitation, 27*(8), 758-767.

Buist-Bouwman, M., Ormel, J., De Graaf, R., Vilagut, G., Alonso, J., Van Sonderen, E., et al. (2008). Psychometric properties of the World Health Organization Disability Assessment Schedule used in the European Study of the Epidemiology of Mental Disorders. *International Journal Of Methods In Psychiatric Research, 17*(4), 185-197.

Chopra, P., Couper, J., & Herrman, H. (2004). The assessment of patients with long-term psychotic disorders: Application of the WHO Disability Assessment Schedule II. *The Australian and New Zealand Journal Of Psychiatry, 38*(9), 753-759.

Commons, T.A., & Lewis, A. J. (2009). Diagnosing borderline personality disorder: Examination of how clinical indicators are used by professionals in the health setting. *Clinical Psychologist, 13*(1), 21-27.

Eddy D. M., & Clanton C. H. (1982). The art of diagnosis: Solving the clinicopathological exercise. *New England Journal of Medicine. 306*(21), 1263-8.

Faison, W. E., & Schultz, S. K. (2011). Diagnostic issues relating to lifespan from adulthood into later life. In The conceptual evolution of DSM-5. American Psychiatric Publishing, Inc. pp. 323-342.

Federici, S. (2010). A note on the theoretical framework of World Health Organization Disability Assessment Schedule II. Disability & Rehabilitation, 32(8), 687-691.

First, M. (2004). Personality disorders conference (December 1-3, 2004). Retrieved October 27, 2013 from: http://www.dsm5.org/Research/Pages/PersonalityDisordersConference(December1-3,2004).aspx?css=print

Frank, E., Rucci, P., & Cassano, G. (2011). One way forward for psychiatric nomenclature: The example of the spectrum project approach. In: *The conceptual evolution of DSM-5*. Washington, D.C. American Psychiatric Publishing, Inc. pp. 37-58.

Gaudiano, B. A., (2013, September 29) Psychotherapy's image problem. *The New York Times*. Retrieved October 27, 2013 from: http://www.nytimes.com

Giguere, A., Labrecque, M., Grad, R., Cauchon, M., Greenway, M., Legare, M., et al. (2012). Barriers and facilitators to implementing decision boxes in primary healthcare teams to facilitate shared decision making: A study protocol. *BMC Medical Informatics & Decision Making, 12*(1), 85-91.

Hays, R. (2009). Development of physical and mental health summary scores from the patient-reported outcomes measurement information system (PROMIS) global items. *Quality Of Life Research, 18*(7), 873-880.

Hu, L., Zang, Y., & Li, N. (2012). The applicability of WHODAS 2.0 in adolescents in China. *Journal Of Clinical Nursing, 21*(17/18), 2438-2451.

Jones, K. (2012). Dimensional and cross-cutting assessment in the DSM-5. *Journal Of Counseling & Development, 90*(4), 481-487.

Kirmayer, L. J., Dandeneau, S., Marshall, E., Phillips, M., & Williamson, K. (2011). Rethinking resilience from indigenous perspectives. *Canadian Journal Of Psychiatry, 56*(2), 84-91.

Krueger, R. F., Eaton, N. R., South, S. C., Clara, L., Simms, L. J. (2011). Empirically derived personality disorder prototypes: Bridging dimensions and categories in DSM-5. In: *The conceptual evolution of DSM-5*. Washington, DC: American Psychiatric Publishing, Inc. pp. 97-118.

Krueger, R. F., Derringer, J., Markon, K. E., Watson, D., & Skodol, A. E. (2012). Initial construction of a maladaptive personality trait model and inventory for DSM-5. *Psychological Medicine, 42*, 1879-1890.

McManamy, J. (2012) Robert Spitzer and the DSM: The most influential psychiatrist you never heard of .http://www.mcmanweb.com/spitzer_dsm.html

Madrid, P., Grant, R., & Rosen, R. (2009). Creating mental health disability through inadequate disaster response: Lessons from Hurricane Katrina. Available from: Gale Virtual Reference Library, Ipswich, MA. Accessed October 23, 2013.

Morey, L. C., Krueger, R. F., Skodol, A. E. (2013). The hierarchical structure of clinician ratings of proposed DSM-5 pathological personality traits. *Journal of Abnormal Psychiatry. 122*(3), 836-41.

Narrow, W. E., Clarke, D. E., Kuramoto, S. J., Kraemer, H. C., Kupfer, D. J., Greiner, L., et al. (2013). DSM-5 field trials in the United States and Canada, part III: Development and reliability testing of a cross-cutting symptom assessment for DSM-5. *American Journal of Psychiatry, 170*, 71-82.

Narrow, W. E., & Kuhl, E. A. (2011). Clinical significance and disorder thresholds in DSM-5: The role of disability and distress. In: *The conceptual evolution of DSM-5*. Washington, DC: American Psychiatric Publishing, Inc. pp. 147-162.

Novak, S. P., Colpe, L. J., Barker, P. R., & Gfroerer, J. C. (2010). Development of a brief mental health impairment scale using a nationally representative sample in the USA. *International Journal Of Methods In Psychiatric Research, 19*, suppl 1, S49-60. doi:10.1002/mpr.313

Prince, M., Glozier, N., Sousa, R., & Dewey, M. (2011). Measuring disability across physical, mental and cognitive disorders. In: *The conceptual evolution of DSM-5*. Washington, DC: American Psychiatric Publishing, Inc. pp. 189-227.

Qing, W., Harris, M. F., Zwar, N., Vagholkar, S., & Campbell, T. (2010). Prerequisites for implementing cardiovascular absolute risk assessment in general practice: A qualitative study of Australian general practitioners' and patients' views. *Journal Of Evaluation In Clinical Practice, 16*(3), 580-584.

Rashed, M. A. (2013). Talking past each other: Conceptual confusion in 'culture' and 'psychopathology'. *South African Journal of Psychiatry, 19*(1), 12-15. doi:10.7196/SAJP.433

Regier, D. A. (2007). Dimensional approaches to psychiatric classification: Refining the research agenda for DSM-5: An introduction. American Psychiatric Institute for Research and Education, *International Journal of Methods in Psychiatric Research 16*(S1): S1–S5 Published online in: Wiley InterScience (www.interscience.wiley.com)

Reiger, D. A. , Narrow, W. E., Kuhl, E. A., & Kupfer, D. J. (Eds.). (2011). *The conceptual evolution of DSM-5*. American Psychiatric Publishing, Washington DC:

Rothstein, D. & Santana, L. (2012). "Make just one change: Teach students to ask their own questions. Cambridge, MA: Harvard Education Press:

Samuel, D. B., Lynam, D. R., Widiger, T. A.,& Ball, S.A. (2012). An expert consensus approach to relating the proposed DSM-5 types and traits. *Personality Disorders, 3*(1), 1-16.

Sapolsky, R. M. (1998). Why zebras don't get ulcers : An updated guide to stress, stress-related diseases, and coping. New York : W.H. Freeman and Co.

Schmeck, K., Schlüter-Müller, S., Foelsch, P. A., & Doering, S. (2013). The role of identity in the DSM-5 classification of personality disorders. *Child & Adolescent Psychiatry & Mental Health, 7*(1), 1-11.

So, J. K. (2008). Somatization as cultural idiom of distress: rethinking mind and body in a multicultural society. *Counselling Psychology Quarterly, 21*(2), 167-174.

Storch, E. A., Khanna, M., Merlo, L. J., Loew, B. A., Franklin, M., Reid, J. M., et al. (2009). Children's Florida obsessive compulsive inventory: Psychometric properties and feasibility of a self-report measure of obsessive–compulsive symptoms in youth. *Child Psychiatry & Human Development, 40*(3), 467-483.

Stumblingbear-Riddle, G., & Romans, J. C. (2012). Resilience among urban American Indian adolescents: Exploration into the role of culture, self-esteem, subjective well-being, and social support. American Indian and Alaska Native Mental Health Research: Centers for American Indian and Alaska Native Health Colorado School of Public Health/University of Colorado Anschutz Medical Campus, *19*(2), 1-19.

Tseng, W., & Streltzer, J. (2008). Cultural Competence in Health Care. New York: Springer.

Üstün, T., Kostanjsek, N., Chatterji, S., and Rehm, J. (Eds.). (2010). Measuring health and disability: Manual for WHO disability assessment schedule WHODAS 2.0. World Health Organization: Geneva, Switzerland.

Üstün, T., Chatterji, S., Kostanjsek, N., Rehm, J., Kennedy, C., Epping-Jordan, J., et al. (2010). Developing the World Health Organization disability assessment schedule 2.0. *Bulletin of the World Health Organization, 88*(11), 815-823.

Verheul, R., (2005). Clinical utility of dimensional models for personality pathology. *Journal of Personality Disorders,* 19, 283-302.

Widiger, T.A., & Simonsen, E. (2005). Alternative dimensional models of personality disorder: finding a common ground. *Personality Disorders, 19*, 110-130.

White, M. & Epston, D. (1990). Narrative means to therapeutic ends. New York: W. W. Norton & Co.

World Health Organization. WHO disability assessment schedule 2.0 WHODAS 2.0. http://www.who.int/classifications/icf/whodasii/en/index.html

Yonkers, K. A., & Clarke, D. E. (2011). Gender and gender-related issues in DSM-5. In The conceptual evolution of DSM-5. American Psychiatric Publishing, Inc. pp. 287-304.

Appendix A

The QFT has six key steps:

Step 1: *Facilitator Designs a Question Focus*. The Question Focus, or QFocus, is a prompt that can be presented in the form of a statement or a visual or aural aid to focus and attract attention and quickly stimulate the formation of questions. The QFocus is different from many traditional prompts, because it is not a leading question. It serves, instead, as the focus for staff questions so staff can, on their own, identify and explore a wide range of themes and ideas. For example, a QFocus for implementing the WHODAS might be: "Mentally ill people are disabled. Disabled people can function autonomously." The staff begin producing questions about what it means to be disabled and what it means to function.

Step 2: *Staff Produce Questions*. Staff use a set of rules that provide a clear protocol for producing questions without assistance from the facilitator. The four rules are: 1) ask as many questions as you can; 2) do not stop to discuss, judge, or answer any of the questions; 3) write down every question exactly as it was stated; and 4) change any statements into questions. Before staff start generating their questions, the facilitator introduces the rules and asks the staff to think about and discuss possible challenges in following them. Once the staff get to work, the rules provide a firm structure for an open-ended thinking process. Staff are able to generate questions and think more broadly than they would have if they had not been guided by the rules.

Step 3: *Staff Improve Their Questions*. Staff then improve their questions by analyzing the differences between open- and closed-ended questions and by practicing changing one type to the other. The facilitator begins this step by introducing definitions of closed- and open-ended questions. The staff use the definitions to categorize the list of questions they have just produced into one of the two categories. Then, the facilitator leads them through a discussion of the advantages and disadvantages of both kinds of questions. To conclude this step, the facilitator asks the staff to change at least one open-ended question into a closed-ended one, and vice versa, which leads staff to think about how the phrasing of a question can affect the depth, quality, and value of the information they will obtain. This step helps to identify barriers and challenges in implementing the changes.

Step 4: *Staff Prioritize Their Questions*. The facilitator, with the goal of implementation in mind, offers criteria or guidelines for the selection of priority questions. For example, the instruction may be, "Choose the three questions you most want to explore further." When designing a pilot, it may be, "Choose three testable questions." During this phase, staff move from thinking divergently to thinking convergently, zero in on the locus of their inquiry, and plan concrete action steps for getting information they need to complete the task.

Step 5: *Staff and Facilitators Decide on Next Steps*. At this stage, staff and facilitators work together to decide how to use the questions. The questions may lead to changes in timeline, responsibility, or administration. Based on the responses, staff may determine what is the most important step or what steps are duplicative.

Step 6: *Staff Reflect on What They Have Learned*. The facilitator reviews the steps and provides staff with an opportunity to review what they have determined by producing, improving, and prioritizing their questions. Making the QFT completely transparent helps staff see what they have done and how it contributed to their conclusions. They can internalize the process and then apply it across settings.

Appendix B

Implementation Checklist for Assessments: Private Practice

Determine practice profile	How many clients What age groups Language(s)
Data collection needs	Use electronically (e.g., download from website) Hand out Mail out
Privacy concerns	HIPAA – Under the recent HIPAA revisions, clients have access to more information. Determine whether you will keep this information or provide it to your clients and only chart the results. Record retention (keep raw data in chart?)
How will you handle sharing results?	Use electronically (e.g., download from website)/ privacy issues Hand out Mail out
Scope of Practice Issues	*Qualification level (see below) that minimally includes formal training in the ethical administration, scoring, and interpretation of clinical assessments
Office Policies/Issues	Add statement in office policies that informs your clients about the purpose and use of the assessments
Coding and Billing Issues	Determine whether you can bill for interpreting the results of the assessments (see scope of practice)

| Forms/Charting | Modify clinical forms (e.g., progress notes) to include results
Make sure forms meet documentation standards (e.g., client name, date of birth, date of service, and client ID at a minimum) |
| Tracking Issues | Determine frequency of administration and how to track |

NOTE: * The DSM-5 does not address qualification levels to administer the assessments available in the hard copy or on its website. The following information is from Pearson Assessments, a leading developer and publisher of psychological assessments, tests, and measures. It is an industry standard of the training needed to administer, score, and interpret clinical assessments and is used to insure that individuals who do not have the minimal background cannot purchase such instruments. It is provided here as a guideline.

Qual A: There are no special qualifications to purchase these products.

Qual B: Tests can be purchased by individuals with:

- Certification by or full active membership in a professional organization (ASHA, AOTA, APA, AERA, ACA, AMA, NASP, NAN, INS) that requires training and experience in a relevant area of assessment.
  OR
- A master's degree in psychology, education, occupational therapy, speech-language pathology, social work, or in a field closely related to the intended use of the assessment, and formal training in the ethical administration, scoring, and interpretation of clinical assessments.

Qual C: Tests with a C qualification require a high level of expertise in test interpretation, and can be purchased by individuals with:

- Licensure or certification to practice in your state in a field related to the purchase.
  OR
- A doctorate degree in psychology, education, or closely related field with formal training in the ethical administration, scoring, and interpretation of clinical assessments related to the intended use of the assessment.

Qual Q: Tests can be purchased by individuals with one of the backgrounds below as determined by the particular purchase, along with formal training in the ethical use, administration, and interpretation of standardized assessment tools and psychometrics:

Q1: A degree or license to practice in the healthcare or allied healthcare field,

OR

Q2: Formal supervised mental health, speech/language, and/or educational training specific to working with parents and assessing children, or formal supervised training in infant and child development

Sample qualified personnel in these categories may include: psychiatrists, early interventionists, social workers, developmental pediatricians, pediatric nurse practitioners, counselors, content or diagnostic education specialists, speech and language therapists, and occupational and physical therapists specializing in early intervention. If you clearly meet the criteria established for B or C levels, you would not need to pursue qualification under Level Q

Appendix C

Implementation Checklist for Assessments: Agency/Group Practice

Determine practice profile	How many clinicians What licenses (see scope of practice below) How many clients What age groups Language(s)
Data collection needs	Use electronically (e.g., download from website) Hand out Mail out
Privacy concerns	HIPAA – Under the recent HIPAA revisions, clients have access to more information. Determine whether you will keep this information or provide it to your clients and only chart the results. Record retention (keep raw data in chart?)
How will you handle sharing results?	Use electronically (e.g., download from website)/privacy issues Hand out Mail out
Scope of Practice Issues	*Qualification level (see below) that minimally includes formal training in the ethical administration, scoring, and interpretation of clinical assessments
Office Policies/Issues	Add statement in office policies that informs your clients about the purpose and use of the assessments

Coding and Billing Issues	Determine whether you can bill for interpreting the results of the assessments (see scope of practice)
Forms/Charting	Modify clinical forms (e.g., progress notes) to include results
Tracking Issues	Determine frequency of administration and how to track
Start Date	Determine when you will start using the assessments Notify all personnel of start date Make note in all charts when this was started Have plan in place to systematically review all current charts to insure documentation is available Have plan in place for all new clients/charts to insure documentation is provided Have plan in place to note for all closed charts that assessments were not being used when the chart was closed.
Policy and Procedure Review	Update all policies regarding data collection and retention Identify key personnel regarding charting, coding and billing, electronic health record (EHR) modification, training
Budget Considerations	Training Written materials Updates to computer code

NOTE: * The DSM-5 does not address qualification levels to administer the assessments available in the hard copy or on its website. The following information is from Pearson Assessments, a leading developer and publisher of psychological assessments, tests, and measures. It is an industry standard of the training needed to administer, score, and interpret clinical assessments and is used to insure that individuals who do not have the minimal background cannot purchase such instruments. It is provided here as a guideline.

Qual A: There are no special qualifications to purchase these products.
Qual B: Tests can be purchased by individuals with:

- Certification by or full active membership in a professional organization (ASHA, AOTA, APA, AERA, ACA, AMA, NASP, NAN, INS) that requires training and experience in a relevant area of assessment.
  OR

- A master's degree in psychology, education, occupational therapy, speech-language pathology, social work, or in a field closely related to the intended use of the assessment, and formal training in the ethical administration, scoring, and interpretation of clinical assessments.

Qual C: Tests with a C qualification require a high level of expertise in test interpretation, and can be purchased by individuals with:

- Licensure or certification to practice in your state in a field related to the purchase.

  OR

- A doctorate degree in psychology, education, or closely related field with formal training in the ethical administration, scoring, and interpretation of clinical assessments related to the intended use of the assessment.

Qual Q: Tests can be purchased by individuals with one of the backgrounds below as determined by the particular purchase, along with formal training in the ethical use, administration, and interpretation of standardized assessment tools and psychometrics:

Q1: A degree or license to practice in the healthcare or allied healthcare field,

OR

Q2: Formal supervised mental health, speech/language, and/or educational training specific to working with parents and assessing children, or formal supervised training in infant and child development

Sample qualified personnel in these categories may include: psychiatrists, early interventionists, social workers, developmental pediatricians, pediatric nurse practitioners, counselors, content or diagnostic education specialists, speech and language therapists, and occupational and physical therapists specializing in early intervention. If you clearly meet the criteria established for B or C levels, you would not need to pursue qualification under Level Q.

Appendix D

Table 1 Level-2 and Severity Specific Screening Measures

Measure Name	Domain	Age Group	Evaluation Period	Administered By	Scoring	Source
LEVEL 2—Depression—Adult	Depression	Adult	Past 7 days	Client	8 questions; 5-point Likert Scale, Summed; higher scores indicate severity	(PROMIS Emotional Distress—Depression—Short Form)
LEVEL 2—Anger—Adult	Anger	Adult	Past 7 days	Client	5 questions; 5-point Likert Scale, Summed; higher scores indicate severity	(PROMIS Emotional Distress—Anger—short Form)
LEVEL 2—Mania—Adult	Mania	Adult	Past 7 days ("past week")	Client	5 questions; 5-point Likert scale (anchor items); higher scores indicate mania; summed raw scores cutoff is 5.	(Altman Self-Rating Mania Scale [ASRM])
LEVEL 2—Anxiety—Adult	Anxiety	Adult	Past 7 days	Client	7 questions; 5-point Likert Scale, Summed; higher scores indicate severity	(PROMIS Emotional Distress—Anxiety—Short Form)
LEVEL 2—Somatic Symptom—Adult	Somatic Sx	Adult	Past two weeks	Client	15 questions; 3-point Likert Scale, Summed; summed scores evaluated on symptom table provided	Patient Health Questionnaire 15 Somatic Symptom Severity Scale [PHQ-15])
LEVEL 2—Sleep Disturbance—Adult	Sleep disturbance	Adult	Past 7 days	Client	8 questions; 5-point Likert Scale, Summed; higher scores indicate severity	(PROMIS—Sleep Disturbance—Short Form)

(Continued)

Table 1 *(Continued)*

Measure Name	Domain	Age Group	Evaluation Period	Administered By	Scoring	Source
LEVEL 2—Repetitive Thoughts and Behaviors—Adult	Repetitive Thoughts	Adult	Past 7 days	Client	5 questions; 5-point Likert Scale, Summed; higher item scores indicate severity; total summed score used to determine cutoff for additional evaluation (≥ 8)	(Adapted from the Florida Obsessive-Compulsive Inventory [FOCI] Severity Scale [Part B])
LEVEL 2—Substance Use—Adult	Substance Use	Adult	Past two weeks	Client	11 items; 5-point Likert Scale; each item rated independently; multiple items rated (≥ 1) indicates severity and complexity	(Adapted from the NIDA-Modified ASSIST)
LEVEL 2—Somatic Symptom—Parent/Guardian of Child Age 6-17	Somatic Sx	Children Ages 6-17	Past 7 days	Parent/Guardian	13 items; 3-point Likert Scale, Summed; higher scores indicate severity	(Patient Health Questionnaire 15 Somatic Symptom Severity Scale [PHQ-15]); two questions omitted because they only apply to adults
LEVEL 2—Sleep Disturbance—Parent/Guardian of Child Age 6-17	Sleep Disturbance	Children Ages 6-17	Past 7 days	Parent/Guardian	8 items; 5-point Likert Scale, Summed; higher scores indicate severity	(PROMIS—Sleep Disturbance—Short Form)

LEVEL 2—Inattention—Parent/Guardian of Child Age 6–17	Inattention	Children Ages 6–17	Past 7 days	Parent/Guardian	8 items; 5-point Likert Scale, Summed; higher scores indicate severity	(Swanson, Nolan, and Pelham, version IV [SNAP-IV])
LEVEL 2—Depression—Parent/Guardian of Child Age 6–17	Depression	Children Ages 6–17	Past 7 days	Parent/Guardian	11 items; 5-point Likert Scale, Summed; higher scores indicate severity	(PROMIS Emotional Distress—Depression—Parent Item Bank)
LEVEL 2—Anger—Parent/Guardian of Child Age 6–17	Anger	Children Ages 6–17	Past 7 days	Parent/Guardian	5 items; 5-point Likert Scale, Summed; higher scores indicate severity	American Psychiatric Association
LEVEL 2—Irritability—Parent/Guardian of Child Age 6–17 (Affective Reactivity Index [ARI])	Irritability	Children Ages 6–17	Past 7 days	Parent/Guardian	7 items; 3-point Likert Scale, Summed; higher scores indicate severity	(PROMIS Emotional Distress—Calibrated Anger Measure—Parent)
LEVEL 2—Mania—Parent/Guardian of Child Age 6–17	Mania	Children Ages 6–17	Past 7 days	Parent/Guardian	5 questions; 5-point Likert scale (anchor items); higher scores indicate mania; summed raw scores cutoff is 5.	(Adapted from the Altman Self-Rating Mania Scale [ASRM])

(Continued)

Table 1 *(Continued)*

Measure Name	Domain	Age Group	Evaluation Period	Administered By	Scoring	Source
LEVEL 2—Anxiety—Parent/Guardian of Child Age 6–17	Anxiety	Children Ages 6-17	Past 7 days	Parent/Guardian	10 items; 5-point Likert Scale, Summed; higher scores indicate severity	(Adapted from PROMIS Emotional Distress—Anxiety—Parent Item Bank)
LEVEL 2—Substance Use—Parent/Guardian of Child Age 6–17	Substance Use	Children Ages 6-17	Past two weeks	Parent/Guardian	11 items; 5-point Likert Scale and a "don't know" (not scored); each item rated independently; multiple items rated (≥ 0) indicates greater severity and complexity	(Adapted from the NIDA-Modified ASSIST)
LEVEL 2—Somatic Symptom—Child Age 11–17	Somatic Sx	Children Ages 11-17	Past 7 days	Client	13 items; 3-point Likert Scale, Summed; higher scores indicate severity	(Patient Health Questionnaire 15 Somatic Symptom Severity Scale [PHQ-15];]; two questions omitted because they only apply to adults)
LEVEL 2—Sleep Disturbance—Child Age 11–17	Sleep Disturbance	Children Ages 11-17	Past 7 days	Client	8 items; 5-point Likert Scale, Summed; higher scores indicate severity	(PROMIS—Sleep Disturbance—Short Form)

LEVEL 2—Depression—Child Age 11–17	Depression	Children Ages 11-17	Past 7 days	Client	8 items; 5-point Likert Scale, Summed; higher scores indicate severity	(PROMIS Emotional Distress—Depression—Pediatric Item Bank)
LEVEL 2—Anger—Child Age 11–17	Anger	Children Ages 11-17	Past 7 days	Client	11 items; 5-point Likert Scale, Summed; higher scores indicate severity	(PROMIS Emotional Distress—Calibrated Anger Measure—Pediatric)
LEVEL 2—Irritability—Child Age 11–17	Irritability	Children Ages 11-17	Past 7 days	Client	5 items; 5-point Likert Scale, Summed; higher scores indicate severity	(Affective Reactivity Index [ARI])
LEVEL 2—Mania—Child Age 11–17	Mania	Children Ages 11-17	Past 7 days	Client	7 items; 3-point Likert Scale, Summed; higher scores indicate severity	(Altman Self-Rating Mania Scale [ASRM])
LEVEL 2—Anxiety—Child Age 11–17	Anxiety	Children Ages 11-17	Past 7 days	Client	5 questions; 5-point Likert scale (anchor items); higher scores indicate mania; summed raw scores cutoff is 5.	(PROMIS Emotional Distress—Anxiety—Pediatric Item Bank)
LEVEL 2—Repetitive Thoughts and Behaviors—Child Age 11–17	Repetitive thoughts	Children Ages 11-17	Past 7 days	Client	10 items; 5-point Likert Scale, Summed; higher scores indicate severity	(Adapted from the Children's Florida Obsessive Compulsive Inventory [CFOCI] Severity Scale)

(Continued)

Table 1 (*Continued*)

Measure Name	Domain	Age Group	Evaluation Period	Administered By	Scoring	Source
LEVEL 2—Substance Use—Child Age 11–17	Substance Use	Children Ages 11-17	Past 7 days	Client	11 items; 5-point Likert Scale and a "don't know" (not scored); each item rated independently; multiple items rated (≥ 0) indicates greater severity and complexity	(Adapted from the NIDA-Modified ASSIST)
Severity Measure for Depression—Adult	Depression	Adult	Past 7 days	Client	9 items; 4-point Likert Scale, Summed; higher scores indicate severity	(Patient Health Questionnaire [PHQ-9])
Severity Measure for Separation Anxiety Disorder—Adult	Separation Anxiety	Adult	Past 7 days	Client	10 items; 5-point Likert Scale, Summed; higher scores indicate severity	American Psychiatric Association
Severity Measure for Specific Phobia—Adult	Specific Phobia Choice of 5 phobic situations – need to use multiple copies if more than one situation is identified by client	Adult	Past 7 days	Client	10 items; 5-point Likert Scale, Summed; higher scores indicate severity;	American Psychiatric Association

Severity Measure for Social Anxiety Disorder (Social Phobia)—Adult	Social Anxiety Disorder	Adult	Past 7 days	Client	10 items; 5-point Likert Scale, Summed; higher scores indicate severity; average total score	American Psychiatric Association
Severity Measure for Panic Disorder—Adult	Panic Disorder	Adult	Past 7 days	Client	10 items; 5-point Likert Scale, Summed; higher scores indicate severity; average total score	American Psychiatric Association
Severity Measure for Agoraphobia—Adult	Agoraphobia	Adult	Past 7 days	Client	10 items; 5-point Likert Scale, Summed; higher scores indicate severity; average total score	American Psychiatric Association
Severity Measure for Generalized Anxiety Disorder—Adult	Generalized Anxiety Disorder	Adult	Past 7 days	Client	10 items; 5-point Likert Scale, Summed; higher scores indicate severity; average total score	American Psychiatric Association
Severity of Posttraumatic Stress Symptoms—Adult	PTSD	Adult	Past 7 days	Client	9 items; 5-point Likert Scale, Summed; higher scores indicate severity; average total score	(National Stressful Events Survey PTSD Short Scale [NSESS])

(*Continued*)

Table 1 (*Continued*)

Measure Name	Domain	Age Group	Evaluation Period	Administered By	Scoring	Source
Severity of Acute Stress Symptoms—Adult	Acute Stress	Adult	Past 7 days	Client	7 items; 5-point Likert Scale, Summed; higher scores indicate severity; average total score	(National Stressful Events Survey Acute Stress Disorder Short Scale [NSESS])
Severity of Dissociative Symptoms—Adult	Dissociative Sx	Adult	Past 7 days	Client	8 items; 5-point Likert Scale, Summed; higher scores indicate severity; average total score	(Brief Dissociative Experiences Scale [DES-B]); DES-B (Dalenberg C, Carlson E, 2010) modified for DSM-5 by C. Dalenberg and E. Carlson.
Severity Measure for Depression—Child	Depression	Children 11-17	Past 7 days	Client	9 items; 5-point Likert Scale, Summed; higher scores indicate severity; average total score	(Patient Health Questionnaire [PHQ-9])
Severity Measure for Separation Anxiety Disorder—Child	Separation Anxiety	Children 11-17	Past 7 days	Client	10 items; 5-point Likert Scale, Summed; higher scores indicate severity; average total score	American Psychiatric Association

Severity Measure for Specific Phobia—Child	Specific Phobia; Choice of 5 phobic situations – need to use multiple copies if more than one situation is identified by client	Children 11-17	Past 7 days	Client	10 items; 5-point Likert Scale, Summed; higher scores indicate severity; average total score	American Psychiatric Association
Severity Measure for Social Anxiety Disorder (Social Phobia)—Child	Social Anxiety Disorder	Children 11-17	Past 7 days	Client	10 items; 5-point Likert Scale, Summed; higher scores indicate severity; average total score	American Psychiatric Association
Severity Measure for Panic Disorder—Child	Panic Disorder	Children 11-17	Past 7 days	Client	10 items; 5-point Likert Scale, Summed; higher scores indicate severity; average total score	American Psychiatric Association
Severity Measure for Agoraphobia—Child	Agoraphobia	Children 11-17	Past 7 days	Client	10 items; 5-point Likert Scale, Summed; higher scores indicate severity; average total score	American Psychiatric Association

(Continued)

Table 1 (*Continued*)

Measure Name	Domain	Age Group	Evaluation Period	Administered By	Scoring	Source
Severity Measure for Generalized Anxiety Disorder—Child	Generalized Anxiety Disorder	Children 11-17	Past 7 days	Client	10 items; 5-point Likert Scale, Summed; higher scores indicate severity; average total score	American Psychiatric Association
Severity of Posttraumatic Stress Symptoms—Child	PTSD	Children 11-17	Past 7 days	Client	9 items; 5-point Likert Scale, Summed; higher scores indicate severity; average total score	(National Stressful Events Survey PTSD Short Scale [NSESS])
Severity of Acute Stress Symptoms—Child	Acute Stress	Children 11-17	Past 7 days	Client	7 items; 5-point Likert Scale, Summed; higher scores indicate severity; average total score	(National Stressful Events Survey Acute Stress Disorder Short Scale [NSESS])
Severity of Dissociative Symptoms—Child	Dissociative Sx	Children 11-17	Past 7 days	Client	8 items; 5-point Likert Scale, Summed; higher scores indicate severity; average total score	(Brief Dissociative Experiences Scale [DES-B]); DES-B (Dalenberg C, Carlson E, 2010) modified for DSM-5 by C. Dalenberg and E. Carlson.

Form A

For free access to all Excel spreadsheets go to *go.pesi.com/DSM-5*.

Level-1 Cross Cutting Symptom Measure Client Feedback Template

Client Name: Client ID: 123456

Date Administered: Clinician:

Thank you for completing the symptom questionnaire. I asked you to complete this so that I might have a better idea of what is bothering you right now. The questionnaire looks at where you may be feeling bothered by symptoms across a broad range of behaviors.

Results are shown below. This is just one way to look at your overall functioning. We will use this, along with other information to determine how best to get your needs met and find appropriate interventions that will help you feel better.

HOW DO I READ THE RESULTS?

Your score is determined by adding together the answers you gave and then noting the most intense level from the questions in each group. Each answer has a value attached to it.

Answer	Value
None (Not at all)	0
Slight (Rare, less than a day or two)	1
Mild (Several days)	2
Moderate (More than half the days)	3
Severe (Nearly every day)	4

If you scored a "0" or a "1", you probably are doing well and do not experience problems in that area.

If you score a "2", you probably are experiencing mild problems and would benefit from some support or assistance.

If you score a "3", you are experiencing moderate problems, and support and assistance should be actively sought.

If you score a "4", your symptoms interfere with your ability to live the kind of life you want and support and assistance are strongly encouraged.

If you score in the mild, moderate, or severe in multiple areas, you may be at higher risk for self-harm, for engaging in behaviors that are unhealthy, or that make you unwell. We will focus on these areas in our work together.

Information contained in this report is protected and confidential. Sharing or use by individuals other than the client or persons not authorized to participate in the treatment of the client is prohibited by federal regulations.

Your Results
CUT AND PASTE EXCEL CHART HERE

What does this mean?
PROVIDE A BRIEF INTERPRETATION OR SUMMARY OF YOUR CLINICAL IMPRESSIONS HERE.

What is the next step?
Schedule an appointment to discuss these results.

Information contained in this report is protecte and confidential. Sharing or use by individuals other than the client or persons not authorized to participate in the treatment of the client is prohibited by federal regulations.

Form B

For free access to all Excel spreadsheets go to *go.pesi.com/DSM-5*.

WHODAS 2.0 Client Feedback Template

Client Name: Client ID:

Date: Clinician Name:

Thank you for completing the WHODAS 2.0. I asked you to complete this so that I might have a better idea of your strengths and the challenges you experience in your daily life. The survey looks at how you manage your life in six very specific domains: understanding and communicating, getting around, self-care, getting along with people, life activities (school/work, and household) and participation in society.

Results are shown below. This is just one way to look at your overall functioning. We will use this, along with other information to determine how best to get your needs met and find appropriate treatment and support for you.

How do I read the results?

Your total score is determined by adding together the answers you gave for a total possible 100 points. Your domain scores are calculated by averaging sum of scores and dividing that by the number of questions in the domain. Each answer has a value attached to it as shown in the chart below.

Answer	Value
None	1
Mild	2
Moderate	3
Severe	4
Extreme/ or Can't Do	5

Domain scores below 2 suggest you probably are doing well and do not experience any disruptive disability in that area.

Domain scores between "2.1" and "3.9" suggest you probably are experiencing **moderate** disability and would benefit from some support or assistance.

Domain scores between "4.0" and "4.9" suggest you definitely are experiencing **severe** disability, and you may be eligible for support and assistance.

A domain score of "5" suggests **extreme** disability or inability and indicates that your disability interferes with your capacity to have a good quality of life. It is likely you would qualify for support and assistance.

If you score in the moderate, severe or extreme range in three or more domains, your quality of life is functionally impaired, and you may qualify for special assistance. Determination of benefits is made by review of this information and extensive documentation of impairment, and cannot be guaranteed solely by completion of this measure.

Your Results
CUT AND PASTE CHART RESULTS FROM EXCEL SHEET HERE.

What does this mean?
PROVIDE A BRIEF INTERPRETATION OR SUMMARY OF YOUR CLINICAL IMPRESSIONS HERE.

What is the next step?
Schedule an appointment to discuss these results. Please remember, this is only a disability screen. To obtain benefits, you must apply.

Determination of eligibility for benefits based on disability is made by review of this and other similar information required by state and federal government regulations. Extensive documentation of impairment is required, and cannot be guaranteed solely by completion of this measure.

Information contained in this report is protected and confidential. Sharing or use by individuals other than the client or persons not authorized to participate in the treatment of the client is prohibited by federal regulations.

Index

Note: Page numbers with *t* indicate tables; those with *n* indicate footnotes.